THE SECRETS OF LONGEVITY

THE SECRETS OF LONGEVITY

S Talalaj and J Talalaj

Hill of Content
Melbourne

First published 1997
by Hill of Content Publishing Pty Ltd
86 Bourke Street, Melbourne 3000

Cover design: Deborah Snibson (The Modern Art Production Group)
Editing and desktop publishing: Bernard Metcalfe (BizWrite Pty Ltd)

National Library of Australia
Cataloguing-in-Publication data

Talalaj, S (Stanislaw), 1923–
The Secrets of Longevity.

Includes index.
ISBN 0 85572 275 4

1. Longevity – Popular works. I. Talalaj, Janusz Joseph.
II. Title

612.68

Author's Note
This book is designed to give current information about recent research into factors affecting the length of human life. While it includes some information related to medical practices, it is not a medical text or reference. The use of information in this book for the purpose of self-treatment without consulting a qualified medical practitioner may be dangerous.

CONTENTS

INTRODUCTION

Early quest for longevity

Since the early history of humanity, there has been an ongoing urge to rejuvenate humans and prolong human life. The ancient approaches to longevity were quite bizarre. In ancient Rome old people sometimes gathered in arenas to drink the fresh blood of dying gladiators. Such blood was said to be the most effective life-prolonging remedy. The belief in the extraordinary properties of human blood was not only confined to ancient Rome; even Pope Innocent III (1161–1216) is said to have drunk the blood of three boys to become young again.

As early as 133 AD, a Chinese alchemist told Emperor Wu-Ti that liquid made from cinnabar (a mercury mineral), and drunk from vessels of gold, would make the drinker immortal. In thirteenth century Europe, it was recognised that many diseases were contagious; it was also generally believed that good health was contagious. Young people who were said to have the greatest amount of health could transmit health to old men and thus reverse the ageing process. In order to accomplish this, an old man had to lie with a young virgin and receive her breath. The practice was first described in the Old Testament (1 Kings 1:1–4), when the servants of King David, an old frail man, said: "Let there be sought for my Lord the King a young virgin; and let her stand before the King and be companion unto him … that the Lord the King may get heat …" This belief survived well into the eighteenth century. For example, a great Dutch physician Boerhaave (1688–1738), advised an old man from Amsterdam to lie between two young girls, assuring him that he would become rejuvenated again.

Some beliefs seem contradictory. On one hand, Taoists in China believe that a man can significantly prolong his life by preventing ejaculation; on the other hand, Australian Aborigines used to administer semen potions to rejuvenate their elderly.

In the 1790s, James Graham made a fortune in London by selling an expensive remedy for prolonging life. He offered Aetherical Ambrosial Quintessence which he manufactured in his special "Adapti-Alchemical Medico-Electrical and Philosophical Apparatus". In addition he employed scantily clad attractive young girls to sell his rejuvenating remedies.

We might be amused by some of these examples, but they show how humans strongly desire a long and healthy life. This book will explore more recent developments in the quest for longevity.

How long do humans live?

In early human history, people lived for only a relatively short time. In ancient Greece for example, the average life expectancy was just 18 years. In ancient Rome it was just 20 years. Nevertheless, long-lived individuals were known in ancient times; Plato, for instance, lived 80 years.

In the 1850s, half the population of the USA died at the age of about 40. At the turn of the twentieth century half the people in the USA survived until 49 years of age. In 1942, Australians and New Zealanders had a life expectancy of 65 years, the highest in the world. Life expectancy at this time was 55 years in Italy while in India it was just 27 years.

Today, life expectancy for white Australians is 76 years for men and 81 for women. The world's highest life expectancy is in Japan, 76.6 years for men and 83 for women. Surprisingly, life expectancy in some developing countries is still quite low. For instance, it is only 43 years in Afghanistan.

In recorded history there have been claims about the incredible longevity of some individuals. The Bible tells us that Methuselah lived 969 years (Genesis 5:27). The Bible also mentions other individuals who lived for hundreds of years.

In 1933, the Chinese press announced that a man born in 1680 had just died in Peking. He was said to have lived 256 years. His supposed date of birth was shown later to be a figment of the imagination.

Exceptional longevity was also reported in the Soviet Union. In the 1950s the Caucasus mountains were said to be home to 500 people aged between 120 and 170. These claims were later found to be false. Dr. Zhores Medvedev, a Russian gerontologist who studied these Russian centenarians, found that they had falsified their birth dates to become famous and gain special State privileges.

Exceptionally long-lived individuals were also said to be found in the Hunza Valley in northern Pakistan, as well as in the Andes region of Equador, but further investigations showed that these reports were also untrue. Currently, the greatest authenticated age to which a human has ever lived is 122 years. The record is held by Jeanne Louise Calment, who, in early 1997, was living in Arles, France.

Chapter One

DIET AND LONGEVITY

Can diet prolong your life to 170 years?

Animal experiments show that diet can prolong life by up to 50 percent. The 'magic' diet is caloric restriction. In essence, caloric restriction means giving much less food than is desired, but ensuring that the diet contains adequate amounts of essential nutrients. Such life extension was first accomplished by Clive McKay who fed one group of rats 60 percent of the calorie intake of a control group. When the normally fed rats were dead, the caloric-restricted rats were still sexually active and showed little sign of ageing or degeneration. Similar results were obtained by investigators in other laboratories. In a human, this would correspond to a life span of about 170 years.

At present it is impossible to say whether caloric restriction could be beneficial to humans but the answer could well be, Yes. So far no one has performed carefully controlled studies over a number of years of the long-term caloric restriction effects in humans. Data obtained from populations who are forced by poverty to live on relatively few calories are uninformative. These diets contain inadequate amounts of essential nutrients. There is, however, some evidence that restricted calorie intake works for the benefit of people who practice it. For example, in Okinawa the local people receive significantly fewer calories than the rest of the Japanese population; they also enjoy only half the national rate of age-related diseases.

Okinawa also boasts the highest proportion of centenarians in Japan. In fact the incidence of centenarians there is up to 40 times greater than that of any other Japanese island. Perhaps, with a better selection of food, these centenarians could have lived even longer.

Caloric restriction can be beneficial even if started at an advanced age. In Madrid, the director of a nursing home, Dr. E. A. Vallejo, put half of his patients on a calorie-restricted diet, alternating 2300 calories with only 800 calories the next day. This dietary programme lasted three years, but the results obtained were truly astounding. The diet-restricted patients had half the incidence of death and half the frequency of infirmary admission when compared to the patients on a normal diet.

Dr. Roy Walford, gerontologist at the University of California Medical School and 'father' of caloric restriction for humans, suggests that 30- to 60-year-old individuals should reduce the daily intake of calories to between 1500 and 2000. One can also accomplish this caloric restriction by intermittent fasting, that is, not eating at all on one, two or three days a week (except water). This programme must be introduced gradually over 5 to 7 years. The amount of calories used would depend on individual build, work performed, medical condition, exercise and similar factors. A middle-aged man should get less than 15 percent of his calories in fats, about 25 percent in protein, and the remainder (60–65%), in complex carbohydrates, vegetables, fruit and grains. As Walford explains, with such low calorie intake it is not possible to choose a combination of food which would provide adequate intake of all necessary nutrients. Thus, when designing our meals, Walford advises us to omit B vitamins and vitamin C and A and zinc from our calculations and take them instead in the form of daily supplements. He argues that one should also take doses of certain vitamins above those officially recommended. This is the case because to maximally prolong the lifespan in rodents, the experimental animals had to be given much larger doses of certain vitamins than could be obtained from their normal diet. As Walford explains: "In transposing the animal data into possible human application, we shall not get far unless we are bold enough to part with Food and Drug Administration (FDA) because we must in some instances considerably exceed a sacred quantity, the Recommended Daily Allowance (RDA)."

Calorie restriction should not be practised from weaning, since a small percentage of calorie-restricted animals die early. Furthermore, it retards growth in rodents.

When calorie restriction was adopted in mid life, a 30 percent prolongation of life was observed in most laboratory rodents. A 50 percent life extension was accomplished by the majority of rats when caloric restriction diet was introduced from weaning. Thus it is advisable not to adopt a caloric restriction diet in humans before the age of 20. All those who intend to switch to such a diet should first consult their medical doctor. Proper diet, however, can significantly extend life even if it does not involve caloric restriction. Many experts estimate that just by choosing appropriate foods you can extend your life expectancy by at least 10 years. In fact, more than 75 percent of people in developed countries eat the wrong foods, substantially increasing the risk of cancer and heart disease. It has been estimated these eating patterns lead to about 35–50% of all cancers.

Does vegetarianism prolong life?

A vegetarian diet leads to human life extension. German researchers at the Cancer Research Centre studied the health of 1904 vegetarians over a period of five years. The results were truly astonishing. These vegetarians had only 37 percent of the number of deaths of the average meat-eating population. The rate of death from cancer was about half the normal rate while for coronary disease the rate was only 20 percent.

British scientists studied 4671 vegetarians for seven years. The death rate from all causes among vegetarians was about

50 percent of the death rate of the general population. For coronary heart disease it was about 40 percent.

In the United States, researchers investigated the link between diet and health in 25,000 Seventh-Day Adventists. These people do not smoke, are teetotallers and about half of them do not eat meat. It has been found that among the Seventh-Day Adventist meat eaters the death rate from coronary heart disease was only 37 percent of the death rate of the average meat-eating population of the United States, while among the Seventh-Day Adventists who were vegetarians it was only 12 percent.

A British study of 1994 involved examining death rates among more than 10,000 people over a period of 12 years, about half of them vegetarians and half meat eaters. It was found that vegetarians, when compared with meat eaters, had a 40 percent lower risk of dying from cancer and 20 percent lower risk of dying from other diseases.

In 1990, scientists showed that a vegetarian diet without the assistance of prescribed medications could be successfully used to retard coronary heart disease (*The Lancet*, 1990). Avoiding meat also helps to prevent diabetes. A study involving 25,000 Americans which lasted 21 years, has shown that people who did not consume meat had only a 45 percent risk of contracting diabetes when compared with the population as a whole. Eating any quantity of meat increased the risk. People who only ate meat once or twice per week had a risk of diabetes 1.4 times that of those who did not eat meat. In those who ate meat six or more times a week the risk increased by 3.8 times.

Some studies found that eating pork more than once a week may double the risk of contracting breast cancer (*British Journal of Cancer*, 1981) and that meat eaters were 2 times more likely to develop gallstones than non-meat eaters (*British Medical Journal*, 1985). In other words, the decision not to eat meat makes a significant difference. More and more people are turning away from meat. Recently it has been found in Britain that about 50 percent of 14–16 year-olds are vegetarians.

Is a vegetarian diet always good for you?

A vegetarian diet may not always be good for you. It may lack some essential nutrients. Although most vegetarians eat a sufficient quantity of proteins, their diet may lack some of the eight essential amino acids. This problem can be resolved, however, by regularly drinking soy milk, eating soy beans or by consuming a wide variety of plant foods. For example, certain amino acids absent in grains are found in legumes. Actually, you do not need to combine various foods in order to get the eight essential amino acids each time you have a meal. What is important is that you get all the essential amino acids in the course of a day.

Some nutritionists maintain that people who refrain from meat and dairy products will have a significant calcium deficiency. This however, need not be the case since leafy vegetables such as broccoli are quite a good source of calcium. In addition, one can consume calcium-fortified foods such as cereals, tofu and orange juice. In fact, vegetarians tend not to have more osteoporosis than meat eaters, or non-meat eaters who consume milk products. This is the case because an excessive protein intake is known to inhibit absorption of calcium. Thus vegetarians who have a lower calcium intake than meat eaters are better able to absorb what they are getting.

Vegetarians however, may have insufficient intake of iron in their diet if they do not eat meat, a rich source of this mineral. Since a low level of iron may lead to anaemia one should ensure that high-iron vegetarian foods are a regular part of one's diet. Dried fruit, pumpkin and sesame seeds are good sources of iron for vegetarians. Iron absorption is facilitated by a sufficient intake of fruits and vegetables containing large amounts of vitamin C.

Vitamin B_{12} is only found in foods of animal origin. Deficiency of vitamin B_{12} can cause pernicious anaemia which can endanger human life. Thus, to avoid deficiency of this vitamin, vegetarians who do not consume dairy products should take vitamin B_{12} supplements. However, some of these vegetarians who do not take supplements have escaped vitamin B_{12} deficiency because they have obtained this vitamin from bacterial contamination of their foods or drinking water. Some amounts of vitamin B_{12} may be found in mushrooms (it comes from the compost in which the mushrooms are grown), and may also be present in fermented soy bean products (produced by the bacteria in such foods). Furthermore, the human liver can store vitamin B_{12} in amounts that can last for five years or longer.

Vegetarians who also abstain from eating eggs and seafood may have a deficiency in zinc, a mineral important to maintenance of good health. Although zinc occurs in many plant foods, its absorption is poor. Eating sufficient amounts of beans, nuts, and various seeds can eliminate this potential deficiency.

Do you need fat in your diet?

Fat contains about twice as much energy per gram as carbohydrates and proteins. Fat provides the body with a store of reserve energy. It is not necessary, however, to consume fat to have it available for storage because both protein and carbohydrates can be converted to fat and stored.

Fats consist of fatty acids combined with glycerol. Although our body can synthesise certain fatty acids, we must obtain others from food. There are three 'essential fatty acids', so called because they are essential for life. Two of them, linoleic and linolenic acids must be obtained from food.

An important group of hormones are made from the essential fatty acids which are involved in the transport of fats within the body. You would receive a sufficient quantity of essential fatty acids even if only a few percent of your total calorie intake were to come from fat. These fatty acids are found in whole grains, seeds and nuts, as well as in fish and meat.

A diet too low in fats would result in a decreased and insufficient intake of fat-soluble vitamins such as vitamins A, D, E and K.

In Australia, the official recommended daily fat intake is in most cases about 40–70 g but it should be less than 31 g according to Walford.

Excessive fat intake has been found to increase the risk of certain types of cancer such as large bowel, pancreatic and hepatic cancers. This is the case because an excess of certain fatty acids found in fats may alter the membrane structure, hence affecting intercellular communication.

Why cholesterol is bad for you

Cholesterol is a well known waxy substance made by the body and also obtained from food. It is not all bad, as it is necessary for production of certain cell components, hormones and important digestive chemicals.

Cholesterol is found principally in meat, butter, cheese and eggs. Other important sources are the saturated fats which are turned into cholesterol within the body. Major sources of saturated fats are animal foods, and palm and coconut oils. Our liver produces the cholesterol our body needs so we do not have to eat animal food. When there is too much cholesterol in the blood it may deposit in the artery walls, narrowing them and leading to a serious disease called atherosclerosis, which may lead to heart attack or stroke.

There are certain proteins to which cholesterol molecules are attached in the bloodstream, namely high density lipoprotein (HDL) and low density lipoprotein (LDL). They are like 'canoes' in which the cholesterol 'passenger' sits. The HDL is not harmful. When the HDL 'canoe' approaches the artery wall, the cholesterol 'passenger' cannot get out of the 'canoe'. In other words, the cholesterol stays in solution within the bloodstream, that is, it does not enter the walls of arteries to form plaque. On the other hand, LDL is harmful because its 'canoe' discharges the cholesterol 'passenger' into the arterial wall where it causes formation of plaque and narrowing of the vessel.

In fact people with elevated serum cholesterol may not have any problems as long as their HDL is also elevated, that is, when the cholesterol/HDL ratio is not higher than 5:1. However, only a small percentage of people have a safe cholesterol/HDL ratio, so that the general rule remains that we should try to keep our blood cholesterol low. Desirable cholesterol levels should be below 5.2 millimoles per litre of blood. At the level of 5.2–6.5 millimoles per litre there is a moderate risk of developing atherosclerosis, but a change of diet may remedy the situation. At cholesterol levels over 6.5 diet alone might not sufficiently reduce the blood cholesterol level. Fortunately efficient cholesterol-lowering drugs are now available.

It was generally assumed until fairly recently that once the plaque was formed inside the artery it could not be removed. We now know that the plaque undergoes a process of exchange with the blood cholesterol. This was demonstrated by applying radioactive cholesterol to patients with advanced atherosclerosis. When such labelled cholesterol was fed it was soon detected being incorporated into the plaque. The same labelled cholesterol could later be detected in the blood again, which proved that cholesterol deposits in the plaque were not permanent. The flow of cholesterol depends on its concentration in the blood. When cholesterol concentration in the blood becomes lower, some cholesterol leaves the plaque and enters the bloodstream, gradually clearing the artery. The plaque becomes thinner, arterial channel is increased and the blood flow is improved. Consequently, atherosclerosis may gradually be reversed so that a bypass operation becomes unnecessary.

Is margarine better than butter?

There is a controversy about the advantage of eating margarine instead of butter. Recent studies link the consumption of margarine with the increased risk of coronary heart disease. Several studies have shown an increased blood cholesterol level in those who regularly eat margarine. The culprits are the so-called trans-fatty acids which promote the formation of cholesterol in the body. These acids are formed during the commercial process of hydrogenation of vegetable oil in the production of margarine. The trans-fatty acid content of margarine is much higher than that of butter. Hard margarine contains about 29 percent of trans-fatty acids. However, butter is infamous for its high saturated fat content, and saturated fats are a source of cholesterol. A partial solution to the problem would be to only consume a type of margarine which is low in the harmful trans-fatty acids, namely to use the so-called soft 'tub' or stick-type margarine. It is best to avoid both butter and margarine and use unprocessed vegetable oils instead.

Do you need sugar?

Although we all like table sugar (sucrose), there is no nutritional reason why we should eat it. It provides us with fuel without any other nutrients such as vitamins or minerals. By eating table sugar we tend to displace more nutritional foods from our diet. Dr. Walford's advice is to eliminate table sugar from your diet.

White sugar is refined to the extent that it no longer contains chromium, an element required for the proper metabolism of glucose. Refined sugar has been linked to hyperactivity in children.

Some studies suggest that excessive sugar consumption may be related to the increased risk of developing coronary heart disease, but these observations have not been confirmed yet. According to surveys carried out in 21 countries, high sugar intake was related to increased breast cancer mortality in women over 30. It is generally assumed that lower sugar intake helps to maintain better health. In fact, people living in the regions where sugar intake is the lowest live much longer and such regions have the highest rates of centenarians.

Sugar has less than half the calories of fat; it has, however, lots of calories packed into a small volume of food. For instance, 30 g of sugar has 109 calories, the same amount as that found in 240 g of apple.

Sugar makes fats more palatable and in this way it further contributes to overeating and obesity. It is estimated that an average Australian consumes about 180 g of sugar daily (65 kg/year). If you are not on a caloric-restriction diet and you love table sugar, try not to exceed 60 g if you are a man or 45 g if you are a woman. It is easy to exceed this level. A typical sugar spoon added to a cup of tea or coffee contains about 8 g of sugar. If you are a woman and you drink just six cups of tea or coffee daily, you already exceed the recommended limit of sugar intake. One soft drink can contains about 40 g of table sugar, while one confectionary bar may contain up to 35 g of table sugar.

Give up sweetening your tea or coffee. Choose unsweetened fruit juice instead of soft drinks full of sugar. And remember that there is plenty of sugar in cakes, biscuits and jams.

Why complex carbohydrates are good for you

Complex carbohydrates are found in all cereals and grain foods, vegetables, potatoes and legumes (lentils, dried beans, peas, etc). A few fruits such as bananas also contain complex carbohydrates. The main sources of complex carbohydrates for people in western countries have been bread and potatoes.

Complex carbohydrates constitute 17 percent of an Australian adult's diet and only 15 percent of an adolescent's. Australian health authorities recommend that complex carbohydrates make up at least 45–50% of our daily calories. Walford argues that they should constitute 60–65% of daily calories for people on caloric restriction. Complex carbohydrates are good sources of vitamins, minerals and dietary fibre.

People consume so few complex carbohydrates because of the myth that they are fattening. Complex carbohydrates provide 4 cal/g. By contrast, proteins contribute 4.3, fats 9, and sugar just 4 cal/g. However, table sugar is not filling so it is easy to take it in large amounts without being aware of it, while complex carbohydrates are usually sufficiently filling so that their consumption is self-limiting in most cases.

To achieve both the official recommended level of complex carbohydrates and the amount recommended by Walford for the caloric restriction diet, an average person would need to eat between 250–300 g of complex carbohydrates daily. One thin slice of bread has 14 g of complex carbohydrates while an average bread roll has 30 g. One cup of cooked pasta contains 40 g of complex carbohydrates, one cup of cooked rice 50 g, and one medium (150 g) potato contains 18 g of complex carbohydrates. Although Walford recommends a higher proportion of complex carbohydrates, he also advocates fewer calories in total so the amounts become roughly the same in each case.

Why too much protein is harmful

Amino acids obtained from animal and plant proteins are used by our body for making the proteins we need. Proteins are used for growth and reproduction of cells, for wound healing and other tissue repair processes. Millions of cells are replaced in the body each second. Amino acids are the building blocks of our hormones, enzymes, antibodies and many other essential components of tissue and blood. In fact, more than 100,000 different body compounds are made from amino acids so that an adequate supply of amino acids is fundamental to our health. Young people need more protein while the elderly need less.

There are 22 amino acids; 14 of them can be manufactured in our body, eight other amino acids must be obtained from food. In Australia, the recommended amount of protein for adults who are moderately active is about 60–110 g daily, while Walford in the caloric restriction diet recommends about 85–115 g of protein daily for 30- to 60-year-olds.

Eating too much protein leads to the excretion in urine of large amounts of minerals. In fact the loss of calcium is directly proportional to the amount of protein consumed. In other words, if you double your intake of protein you will lose 50 percent more calcium by excreting it in urine. It has been found that many people have a negative mineral balance because of the excess of protein they eat. It has been estimated that an adult's protein intake of 225 g per day will lead to a 4 percent skeleton loss per year, even if the calcium intake was 1400 mg daily.

Excessive regular intake of protein may be hazardous. According to a study conducted by the CSIRO Division of Human Nutrition in Adelaide in 1986, high protein intake may increase the risk of stomach cancer. The proteins become incompletely digested and irritate the gastrointestinal tract which, according to some researchers, may lead to malignant growth. Diet with excessive protein intake can also be harmful to kidneys because the nitrogen which is produced from proteins puts considerable stress on kidneys and may impair their function.

It is, however, important to consume a variety of foods containing proteins to get a sufficient supply of all necessary amino acids. Wholemeal bread is a rich source of the essential amino acids. Soy is also an excellent source of proteins. It is one of the few plant foods that give, in required balance, the eight essential amino acids which cannot be produced by our body. One cup of soy beans (200 g) supplies 34 g of protein. Thus 2–2.5 cups of mature soy beans will satisfy the daily protein needs for an adult. Meat is a well-known source of all essential amino acids but vegetarians as a group appear to be in better general health than meat eaters, although this may be due to other lifestyle factors such as exercise.

How good is the Scarsdale diet?

The Scarsdale diet is the brainchild of Dr. Herman Tarnower. His diet would comprise 43 percent protein, 22.5 percent fat and 34.5 percent carbohydrates. For the first two weeks an individual is asked to limit caloric intake to just 1000 cal daily.

Then one is allowed to increase the intake to 1500–1700 cal depending on body size. However, when you get 4 pounds above a certain weight, regarded by Dr. Tarnower as appropriate to your sex and height, you return to the 1000 calorie diet until you shed the 4 pounds.

While the idea of a significant caloric restriction is sound, the recommended amount of protein and fat in this diet is too high. Although a high protein intake is beneficial in childhood it is harmful in later life, particularly for the elderly. The suggested daily intake of fat in this diet is also harmful. It is a well established fact that the best results in increasing the lifespan of experimental animals were achieved when the calorie-restricted diet contained less than 15 percent fat. Over 30 percent fat intake in the Scarsdale diet is hazardous as it may lead to elevated blood cholesterol levels and result in atherosclerosis. So this diet may contribute to life shortening and therefore should not be recommended.

Can Pritikin's diet prolong your life?

Nathan Pritikin claimed that his new diet was "probably the most feasible method of obtaining an extra 20–30 years of vigorous life." He maintained that his diet was the most healthy diet and that it could prevent a number of diseases, especially in the elderly, including coronary heart disease and diabetes.

There is no caloric restriction involved but Pritikin's diet differs from the typical Western diet in that 80 percent of the calories come from complex carbohydrates, and only about 10 percent from both protein and fat. Furthermore, Pritikin prohibits taking refined sugar and table salt. He suggests that one should not drink alcohol, refrain from drinking coffee and should stop smoking. Pritikin's diet consists mainly of various grain products with plenty of fruit and vegetables.

Pritikin's diet, which is low in fat, may be beneficial to those who are trying to control or lose weight. This diet will also significantly reduce blood cholesterol level.

The Pritikin diet resembles the diet recommended by the American Heart Association, so that it can be beneficial to your heart and hence prolong your life. However, unlike Walford's caloric restriction diet, it does not help prevent other major diseases and hence it would probably not extend life to the degree that caloric restriction would.

Why Dr. Atkins' diet is bad for you

Dr. Atkins' prescription for substantial weight loss is unlimited amounts of saturated fats and cholesterol-rich foods, but few carbohydrates.

With too low consumption of carbohydrates, fats are not properly burnt and highly toxic ketons form. Ketons significantly reduce appetite and have been shown to lead to short-term weight loss. However, no controlled studies have been carried out to support the claim that such a diet will lead to long-term weight loss. This diet is particularly hazardous to diabetic patients as it may lead to coma and death.

An unlimited intake of saturated fats and cholesterol-loaded foods advocated by Dr. Atkins leads to substantially increased risk of coronary heart disease. Thus, it is a life-shortening diet. Small wonder that this diet has been condemned by the National Health and Medical Research Council of Australia.

Do you need salt?

Although salt is essential to maintain normal blood pressure, its excessive use is harmful. It is in fact the most important dietary factor linked with high blood pressure, which predisposes to stroke.

Researchers who examined the stroke rate in various countries found that it is strongly related to average salt intake. The lowest level of strokes was observed in regions where the average daily salt intake was the lowest.

Australia and other Western countries have a stroke rate 100 times higher than Papua New Guinea. High dietary salt intake leads to an increase in blood pressure, putting more pressure on the heart muscle and the whole artery system. Too high a salt consumption can have adverse affects on kidneys, causing water retention and swelling of tissues. Excessive salt intake is also hazardous to asthmatics because sodium, the main salt component, makes the air passage in the lungs more sensitive to various irritants.

High salt intake also has a negative impact on the balance of calcium—the more salt you eat, the more calcium is excreted.

According to H. Vottarbee of Louisiana State University Medical Center, Americans eat 15 g of salt daily in their food, while for optimum health 1 scant teaspoon of 4–5 g of salt daily is the required amount. Elimination of the use of table salt may not be the solution to the problem. In a Western diet most salt consumed is obtained from processed foods. The major source of salt in our food is red meat (30–38%) and cereal products (27–28%), which together constitute about 60 percent of total salt intake. It is easy to exceed the recommended salt level intake. Just one hamburger has 1.2 g of sodium.

Salt substitutes can be hazardous for anyone with kidney impairment. Furthermore, some salt substitutes can still contain 50 percent salt. Vegetable salts are based on salt and they will not lower your blood pressure.

Can water extend your lifespan?

A large intake of water can be helpful in prolonging your life. This can be accomplished because water is the perfect aid to weight control and to maintaining good health. Water does not supply us with calories, it suppresses appetite and helps in metabolising fat. When you do not drink sufficient water your kidneys cannot eliminate impurities efficiently or break down stored fat into useable energy. As a result, more fat is stored in your body. Drinking a sufficient amount of water reverses this process. In fact, dehydration is believed to be one of the causes of accelerated ageing. Young, healthy skin loses a lot of water which must be replaced, otherwise skin becomes wrinkled.

Even brain cells are affected by dehydration which causes upset of the hormone balance. For this reason gerontologists recommend that with increasing age there must be a gradual increase in water intake to slow down senescence. An average human being loses about 3 litres of water every day as a result of excretion and perspiration and it is of utmost importance to replace it. At least 2 litres of water daily should be taken in the form of a drink, the rest could come from food.

The best source of water is water itself. Many beverages act as diuretics and they promote a loss of water despite high intake. In particular, the intake of a large amount of alcohol causes an excessive loss of water which must be replaced. This is why those who drink alcohol are advised to drink at least one glass of water with each alcoholic drink. Coffee, and tea and various caffeine-containing drinks are also strong diuretics. Soft drinks, despite their popularity, cannot be considered a perfect source of water because they usually contain excessive amounts of sugar. And a high sugar intake is not considered to be healthy.

Water is a good source of important minerals such as magnesium, selenium and calcium. The link between the water constituents and the incidence of cardiovascular diseases has been observed in many regions of the world including Japan, Sweden, USA and England. In the areas where people drank soft water deficient in such minerals as magnesium and calcium, there was a greater incidence of heart disease and hardening of arteries. On the other hand, in the areas where people drank so-called hard water, that is water rich in minerals, there was a much lower incidence of these diseases. In fact the softer the water you drink, the higher the incidence of heart attacks and the risk of increased mortality.

In some regions, including Australia, it is customary to use rain water for drinking because it is regarded as better than the general water supply. However, this is not the best option as rain water is typically soft water and its use must be considered hazardous, even if the possibility that the rain water may be contaminated with bacteria is ignored. A water supply experiment was performed in Monroe County, Florida, USA. The rain water supply was changed to deep well water so that the water hardness (measured by the quantity of minerals in the water), increased from 0.5 parts per million to hardness levels 400 times greater. It was found that within four years there was a considerable difference in the health of local inhabitants. In fact, the death rate from coronary heart disease dropped from the 500–700 range to 200–300 per 100,000. Thus, if your tap water is soft it is advisable to purchase spring water for drinking.

Drinking water may be contaminated by lead from old pipes or may contain an excessive amount of harmful chlorine. A good home filtering system is recommended to avoid these contaminations. It must be properly maintained however, because an uncleaned water filter may become a source of harmful bacteria.

Chapter Two

LONGEVITY AGENTS IN FOOD

Ascorbic acid

Ascorbic acid (vitamin C) is found in citrus fruits, strawberry, cabbage, brussels sprouts, broccoli, kiwi fruit, peppers and various leafy vegetables. Ascorbic acid is among the most important vitamins involved in the control of harmful free radicals within the body. Free radicals play an important role by promoting oxidation that produces energy. In excess, however, they are harmful because they can damage cell wall and cell content, thus contributing to various diseases and accelerating the ageing process.

Vitamin C, together with vitamin E and beta carotene, is among the strong free radical scavengers—also called antioxidants.

It is has been revealed that laboratory animals fed food containing large amounts of antioxidants tend to live longer. Increased lifespan was observed in various rodents, nematodes and fruit flies when these animals were given large amounts of antioxidants in their diet. In mice, an increased lifespan of up to 30 percent could be observed.

Vitamin C may also help to prevent coronary heart disease in humans. It acts by preventing the formation of atherosclerotic plaque. Researchers at the University of California investigated the relationship between the death rate and vitamin C intake in some 11,000 men and women. They found a significant decline in the death rate from heart attack in those who had a high vitamin C intake. Several studies suggest that vitamin C may also help protect against certain forms of cancer, especially lung, breast and pancreatic cancer.

The FDA's Recommended Daily Allowance for vitamin C is 60 mg. However, a tobacco smoker requires more than 250 mg of vitamin C daily to have the same blood concentration of this vitamin as a non-smoker who takes 60 mg daily. Walford advises non-smokers to take 200 mg of vitamin C daily.

Vitamin C is best obtained from fresh fruit and vegetables because cooking and prolonged storage destroys most of this vitamin. Dried fruit contains little vitamin C. Vegetables kept hot for half an hour or more after cooking may lose more than 75 percent of their vitamin C. Freezing, however, has no depleting effect on this vitamin.

Beta carotene

Beta carotene is the pigment that makes carrots, pumpkins, apricots and rock melon orange. It is also found in green vegetables. Beta carotene is the precursor of vitamin A and is a free radical scavenger.

A study performed at the Harvard University Medical School in 1992 showed that beta carotene may significantly reduce the risk of heart attack. Over a period of six years researchers administered beta carotene supplement to 333 men with symptoms of coronary heart disease. The men who received beta carotene had half as many heart attacks as the control group. In addition, many studies suggest that beta carotene may protect against certain forms of cancer.

The officially recommended dose of beta carotene is 3 mg daily but some gerontologists suggest that one should take about 6 mg of beta carotene daily either from food or as supplements.

High doses of beta carotene may cause serious side effects if taken with large amounts of alcohol. It has been found that baboons given large amounts of alcohol plus 30 mg of beta carotene daily had more severe liver damage than those who received alcohol alone. At present we do not know what precisely is the safe upper limit of alcohol that can be taken with beta carotene supplements. According to Dr. Kenneth Cooper it should be no more than about two beers or two average-sized 4-ounce glasses of wine. He also recommends that you take beta carotene supplement at least four hours before or after you drink alcohol. A large intake of beta carotene supplements can also be hazardous if you are a heavy smoker.

Citrus fruits

Citrus fruits such as orange, lemon and grapefruit seem to be especially created for the benefit of elderly people. These fruits not only contain large amounts of valuable vitamin C which is a potent free radical scavenger, but also other valuable substances such as bioflavonoids and coumarins. Bioflavonoids show strong antioxidant action and help prevent cell damage caused by free radicals. In this way bioflavonoids may help prevent coronary heart disease and delay the symptoms of ageing. Coumarins decrease blood coagulation and prevent the formation of dangerous clots which may cause heart attack and stroke.

Even pectins found in the pulpy membranes of citrus fruit are beneficial to our health. Researchers at the University of Florida College of Medicine have revealed that pectins obtained from grapefruit can reduce blood cholesterol levels by about 7.6 percent, and hence reduce the risk of developing atherosclerosis.

There is some scientific evidence that eating large amounts of various citrus fruits can be beneficial in cancer prevention. A study performed recently in Sweden showed that people who eat citrus fruit on a daily basis had a significantly reduced risk of pancreatic cancer. Research has also shown that a diet rich in citrus fruit may delay the formation of malignant cells. This was demonstrated when cancer-causing chemicals were given to experimental animals together with a diet rich in citrus fruit.

It has recently been found that citrus fruits also contain an anticancer substance in its 'skin' which is removed before eating. A substance called limonene isolated from the fruit skin was found to have an anticancer action. When this compound was given to rats with chemically induced cancer, shrinking of the tumours could be observed. Research will show whether this compound may become a useful anticancer agent in humans.

Cruciferous vegetables

Cruciferous vegetables include broccoli, cabbage, cauliflower and kale. Recent studies have shown that these vegetables are helpful in preventing cancer. The research team at Johns Hopkins University School of Medicine has established that cruciferous vegetables contain a cancer-fighting compound called sulforaphane. This substance was shown to stimulate body cells to produce special enzymes which inhibit cancer growth. Although sulforaphane is found mainly in cruciferous vegetables, it occurs also in carrots, onions and brussels sprouts.

There is some evidence that men who eat a lot of cruciferous vegetables have a much lower risk of developing colon cancer.

Ellagic acid

Ellagic acid is a substance which occurs in a number of fruits. Strawberries, grapes and cherries are a good source of ellagic acid. This compound was studied by Japanese researchers who were the first to discover its anticancer action. Experimental rats were first given a potent chemical substance inducing tumour of the tongue and were then fed a diet rich in ellagic acid. All these rats remained healthy, in contrast to the control group which developed cancer.

In another study, the effect of ellagic acid on a nicotine-derived carcinogen found in cigarette smoke was examined in animal cells. This study showed that ellagic acid, as well as other related polyphenolic substances, reduced the carcinogenic effects of nicotine in experimental animals. Extensive research is required to determine if ellagic acid can be of benefit to humans as a cancer-preventing remedy. Nevertheless it would probably be wise to keep this evidence in mind when selecting your food.

Fibre

There is a group of foods that prevent or at least delay 17 ailments: colorectal cancer, atherosclerosis, diabetes, constipation, haemorrhoids, irritable bowel, diverticulosis, appendicitis, gallstones, hiatus hernia, varicose veins, obesity, gout, high blood pressure, elevated cholesterol level and osteoarthritis.

The miraculous food is dietary fibre. Unfortunately, until recent times people in the West either ignored fibre or tried at least to eliminate it from food products. The reasoning seemed to be correct. After all, fibres are the indigestible remnants of plant foods left over after the gut has absorbed everything we need. Why bother with fibre which has no essential nutrients, minerals or vitamins?

The beneficial value of fibre for our health was first noted by Dr. Denis Burkitt in the 1960s. After his long studies he found that the diseases listed above were much less common in developing countries than in the West. In fact he noted that coronary heart disease, atherosclerosis, and high blood pressure, as well as bowel cancer, were practically unknown in many parts of Africa and Asia. Thus he concluded that people's diet was the key.

People in the West reduced their fibre intake by 80 percent by decreasing consumption of starch and cereals, and by turning to white flour, sugar, fat and red meat. On the other hand, people in developing countries eat little of these 'civilised' foods unless they move to the city where they suffer from the same incidence of these diseases as we do.

Lignin, which occurs in fibre found in root vegetables and cereals, binds bile acids which are made from cholesterol. Consequently, these bile acids become unavailable so the body must convert even more cholesterol into bile acids. Thus, less cholesterol becomes available to clog up arteries. Pectins and gums found in the fibre of various fruits and legumes can also significantly reduce the amount of blood cholesterol. In addition, pectins reduce the blood sugar and so less insulin is produced by the pancreas. In this way pectins may at least delay the onset of diabetes. But probably the most important value of fibre is its protective effect against constipation. Chronic constipation may lead to haemorrhoids and varicose veins. In fact, sufficient fibre in a diet acts like a sponge in the bowel, drawing water into faeces and making the stool softer and easier to pass. Soft stools move quicker down and out of the gut, causing less pressure on the bowel wall and decreasing the risk of constipation. High fibre in the diet may even prevent colorectal cancer. According to a report of the National Cancer Institute (USA), it has been estimated that if fibre intake was increased to 30 g daily, the rate of colorectal cancer would be dramatically reduced.

You should consume between 30–40 g of fibre with your food every day. However, do not overdo it. Too large a dose of fibre may cause diarrhoea and flatulence. A person adopting a fibre-rich diet should increase their intake gradually. When your stools become soft and you no longer experience constipation then you should maintain your fibre intake at that level.

Excessive fibre intake may have some adverse effects. Because of rapid transit time of the bowel contents due to high fibre intake, certain important minerals such as iron, calcium, magnesium, and zinc may leave the body with the stools.

Folic acid

Folic acid (also known as folacin) is an essential vitamin of the B group which is necessary for the synthesis of DNA and thus the formation of new cells. Low levels of folic acid are related to some serious diseases. According to a study at Bringham Hospital in Boston which included 26,000 men and women, those who had the lowest intake of folic acid were found to have the highest level of precancerous tumours of the colon and rectum. The researchers believe that the deficiency of folic acid may initiate tumour formation by allowing cancer-inducing genes to be expressed. Researchers at the University of Alabama have found that women with the highest level of folacin had the lowest level of abnormal cell growth of the cervix even when they were infected with human papilloma virus. The researchers point out that folic acid may provide some protection against this potentially lethal virus.

Folic acid deficiency due to inappropriate diet is widespread among the elderly. It has been found that in England about one person in seven over the age of 70 has some degree of folacin deficiency. As a result of such a deficiency red blood cells become enlarged and their oxygen-carrying capacity is reduced. This causes anaemia which triggers various symptoms such as fatigue, irritability and forgetfulness.

Folacin deficiency can be prevented by eating large amounts of fresh green vegetables such as lettuce, broccoli and spinach, and by eating yeast products.

Folic acid can be readily destroyed by prolonged cooking. Up to 90 percent of folic acid may be lost in this way. Although milk is a good source of folic acid, up to 80 percent of it can be destroyed by pasteurisation.

Green tea

For a long time epidemiologists have been puzzled why men in Japan, who are among the heaviest smokers, have such a low rate of lung cancer. It was hypothesised that widespread drinking of green tea could be the reason, simply because this type of tea is rarely consumed in Western countries. Further observations have revealed that in central Japan where green tea consumption is at its highest, the rate of lung cancer is the lowest. In addition, a survey has shown that Japanese who drink 4–6 cups of green tea daily have a much lower incidence of breast, liver, pancreatic and skin cancer than people who drink less green tea or none at all.

The anticancer action of green tea has recently been investigated by the American Health Foundation in New York. A group of mice was first exposed to cancer-inducing tobacco smoke and then treated with green tea extract. About 45 percent fewer cancers were observed in treated animals when compared with the control group of animals. Green tea differs from ordinary tea in that it is less vigorously processed so it retains some medicinally valuable substances which are lost during the fermentation process of Western teas. From the leaves of green tea Japanese scientists isolated epigallocatechin gallate (EGCG), the compound which is said to be a cancer-suppressing agent. According to the *Japanese Journal of Clinical Oncology* (1993), EGCG inhibits tumour growth in experimental animals. They explain that it inhibits the activity of a tumour promoter called teleocidin and in this way suppresses the malignant growth.

Lycopene

Lycopene is a carotenoid pigment which gives some fruits their reddish colour. It is mainly found in tomatoes, ruby red grapefruit and red pepper. Recent studies have shown that low levels of lycopene in the body can be associated with an increased risk of cancer of the pancreas. According to a study performed at Johns Hopkins University, people suffering from cancer of the pancreas have a much lower level of lycopene in their blood than healthy individuals. In fact, those who had the lowest blood lycopene were found to have more than a five times higher risk of pancreatic cancer when compared with healthy individuals with the highest lycopene levels.

These results are important because pancreatic cancer is often fatal. Although there is still insufficient evidence to demonstrate that a diet rich in lycopene can prevent the development of pancreatic cancer, it is better to be on the safe side and consume large quantities of tomatoes and other fruits containing lycopene.

Perillyl alcohol

Perillyl alcohol, a compound isolated from cherries, has been shown to be active against various cancers in experimental animals. According to Pamela Cromwell from Indiana University School of Medicine, Indianapolis, perillyl alcohol may be regarded as a potential cancer-preventing agent. Cromwell, who performed her studies on rodents, is at present studying the cancer-suppressing effects of this compound on isolated cancer cells. She found that perillyl alcohol inhibits cell contacts in cultures of human pancreatic tumour cells and by this action it slows down tumour growth. The results of this encouraging study have been published in the *Journal of the American Medical Association (JAMA)* (1995).

Researchers and other medical centres are undertaking similar studies in order to explain the mechanism of this cancer suppressing effect of perillyl alcohol. First clinical trials have recently commenced at the University of Iowa College of Medicine, Iowa City.

Proanthocyanidins

Proanthocyanidins, also known as pycnogenols, are a type of bioflavonoids which occur in many fruits and vegetables. Researchers of the Nagasaki University of Medicine in Japan have established that these compounds are strong free radical scavengers, more potent than vitamin C and E.

The first preparations containing proanthocyanidins were obtained in France from the substances isolated from the bark and needles of the pine tree. They are now produced on a commercial scale from grape seeds. This new medicine has become popular in France and other European countries. It is now available in capsule form in Australia.

The producers of the medicine claim the grape seed extract can help cure a number of diseases including coronary heart disease and cancer. Some pamphlets attached to the product claim that this new medicine can cure over 20 different ailments.

The producers of the remedy admit that pycnogenols may be found in fruit and vegetables we consume daily especially in cranberries and cola nuts, but they explain that the content of these flavonoids is extremely low because of the damage caused by improper storage. They say "modern methods of freezing, canning and cooking can have a catastrophic effect. The marvellous nutrients so highly concentrated in pycnogenols are especially hit by modern technology, which has the effect of seriously denaturing it."

Selenium

Although we only require a small amount of selenium in our daily diet, it has so many important functions that its deficiency may be associated with various ailments. Selenium appears to have a protective effect against coronary heart disease and stroke. It has been demonstrated that in the American States in which the selenium level in the soil is the highest, the rate of cancer is the lowest. Thus a low blood selenium level may contribute to the development of cancer.

Researchers believe that selenium supplements may become a useful cancer-prevention program. In one such trial conducted in China people living in a region with a high incidence of stomach cancer were given selenium in their diet. This resulted in a substantial decrease in the rates of stomach cancer when compared with a control group which received placebo. A recent study carried out in the US involved 1500 men and monitored the effect of selenium intake on the rate of prostate cancer. A reduction of more than 50 percent in the incidence of prostate cancer was observed in the group which regularly took selenium supplement when compared with the group which received placebo. These results confirm previous suggestions that a high selenium diet may be useful in preventing development of prostate cancer. The officially recommended level is 50–100 mcg daily. Walford recommends 150 mcg.

Selenium occurs in a variety of foods especially in wholemeal bread. Just 100 g of such bread daily may supply us with 60 mcg of this mineral. Other good sources of selenium include sesame seeds, garlic, onions, broccoli, red grapes and mushrooms, but the selenium level varies with its content in the local soil. People who regularly take selenium supplements should take care not to exceed 300 mcg daily because higher levels can be toxic.

Soy

Recent studies performed in Japan and other countries have shown that soy may be considered a protective agent against cancer. Studies have revealed that women who consumed large amounts of soy milk or other soy-based products, had a significantly lower risk of developing breast cancer. This relationship was especially evident among the Japanese women whose diet included a variety of soy bean products. A survey conducted in China and Singapore has revealed that those women who had breast cancer had consumed much less soy food that those women who remained healthy.

These observations have been confirmed by another study. It has been found that certain substances isolated from soy show anti-tumour effects. These substances inhibit the activity of a certain enzyme that can induce malignant growth. This enzyme inhibitor is called the Bowman-Birk Inhibitor (BBI) and its tumour-suppressing action has been demonstrated in animal trials. When a group of rats was given carcinogens causing colon cancer, treating them with BBI prevented development of cancer in all animals treated. Similar anticancer effects were observed with liver cancer-inducing chemicals.

Genistein, another substance isolated from soy, was also found to have an anticancer effect. In a test-tube experiment with isolated cells it has been shown that genistein inhibits growth of the prostate cancer cells. Further studies in humans will show whether soy can be helpful in preventing cancer.

According to a study performed at the University of Kentucky, Lexington, diet rich in soy proteins can lower blood cholesterol levels. "People with the highest level of cholesterol benefited the most from eating soy protein," says Dr. J. W. Anderson, who conducted the study. In another study reported in the *New England Journal of Medicine* (1995), volunteers who consumed half their proteins from soy had their blood cholesterol lowered by about 10 percent. Some studies indicate that apart from a general reduction in blood cholesterol the soy-rich diet is beneficial because it reduces the blood level of LDL (low density lipoprotein) linked to the development of atherosclerosis.

Tocopherol

Tocopheral (vitamin E) is often called the vitamin of youth. Recent studies have shown that regular intake of this vitamin may not only help prevent some diseases but it may also retard the ageing process. In fact, individuals with a deficiency of vitamin E in their diet display an elevated number of dark brown spots on the skin which increase with age. Animal experiments seem to confirm that vitamin E supplements may extend the animal's life expectancy. A recent study at Harvard University (1993) revealed that 40,000 males who regularly took vitamin E supplements had a 40 percent decreased risk of developing coronary heart disease. Similar studies involved 87 female nurses who were monitored for eight years. Those who consumed high amounts of vitamin E supplements in their diet had the lowest risk of coronary heart disease.

Low levels of vitamin E intake have been linked to the risk of developing lung cancer. A study performed at the Johns Hopkins School of Hygiene and Public Health showed that individuals with the lowest blood levels of vitamin E had the highest incidence of lung cancer.

The beneficial effects of vitamin E are related to its antioxidant properties. As a free radical scavenger vitamin E fights free radicals before they can damage the vital parts of the cells. Experiments have shown that in rats with vitamin E deficiency, age pigments accumulate in the muscles and the uterus. This is why vitamin E is now acquiring the status of an 'anti-ageing' vitamin.

Although deficiency in vitamin E is rare, some doctors prescribe vitamin E to their patients, especially those with potential coronary heart disease. Vitamin E is found in vegetable oils, meat, leafy greens, wheat germ and nuts. Megadoses of vitamin E, of about 3200 IU per day, may be hazardous and should be avoided. They may cause serious side effects, including blurred vision and elevated blood pressure. They may also cause a decrease in thyroid hormone levels. Excessive vitamin E doses are particularly hazardous in people who are treated with anticoagulant drugs.

The recommended daily allowance for vitamin E is about 10 IU but a number of gerontologists recommend a daily dose of up to 600 IU.

Umbelliferous vegetables

Vegetables obtained from the *Umbelliferae* plant family such as carrot, parsnip and celery have been shown to contain a number of substances which might be helpful in preventing cancer. Research conducted at the National Cancer Institute in the United States reveals that certain substances which occur in these vegetables inhibit the initiation of malignant growths in experimental animals. These substances belong to various chemical groups and include carotenoids, flavonoids, and coumarins. In addition, all these groups of substances occurring in fresh vegetables are free radical scavengers; thus they reduce the risk of developing coronary heart disease.

Zinc

Zinc is essential for many enzymes to function and it also regulates their activity within cells. It has a role in the synthesis of proteins and the building blocks of DNA, and helps maintain the structural integrity of some large proteins such as insulin.

An adult human body contains about 1800 mg of zinc. The highest concentrations of this mineral are found in the pigmented membrane of the eye and in the prostate gland. Although scientists have not clearly established what the role of zinc is in these tissues, we know that a cancerous prostate gland contains only one-third as much zinc as a normal one. It has been found that in regions where the elderly eat food rich in zinc there are fewer prostate cancers.

Zinc deficiency and/or low diet intakes have been reported in many countries including the USA, Canada, Sweden and the UK. Its deficiency is associated with hardening of the arteries. Zinc helps to neutralise the toxic mineral cadmium, high intake of which is linked to heart disease.

The symptoms of strong zinc deficiency include mental disturbances, retarded growth in children, and degeneration of the testicles leading to impotence.

The recommended daily intake of zinc for adults and for children over 12 years is 12 mg. Zinc deficiency can occur in people who have inadequate diet; it occurs in some elderly people. Drinking excessive alcohol leads to considerable loss of zinc in the urine, so heavy drinkers often develop zinc deficiency even if they have a proper diet. Doses of zinc above 150 mg daily are toxic.

Chapter Three

LIFESTYLE AND LONGEVITY

Can having a spouse extend your lifespan?

There is sufficient evidence to maintain that married people, regardless of their race, live longer than those who are single, widowed or divorced.

According to a Brazilian study, the mortality rate of single men aged 30–39 in Sao Paulo is ten times higher than that of married men. It is also significantly greater for solitary men of other ages, as well as for women. Thus the researchers conclude that "marriage can be an excellent remedy for longevity." Studies in the western countries also show that married people live longer.

We still do not know for sure how marriage may promote longevity. Perhaps those who are married have better diet, and better care and medical aid when ill. Frequency of sexual intercourse per week was also found to be among important factors linked with longer life.

Being single may be a source of harmful stress since, according to our social norms, married life is considered to be ideal; this may explain why single people have a shorter life expectancy. Losing one's spouse as a result of sudden death or divorce, after many years of living in harmony together, may also contribute to shortened life expectancy due to the considerable stress involved.

Can pet ownership prolong your life?

Pets can enhance the health of their owners. We now find cats and dogs in hospitals, old people's homes, in schools for handicapped children and in some drug addiction units. As Professor Samuel Corson of Ohio State University explains, "Seriously ill people who play with cats or other pets become different people; they receive the kind of love which helps the most." This assumption has been confirmed by many studies. In 1992, a study of the health condition of 5700 pet and non pet-owners was conducted by the Baker Medical Research Institute in Melbourne. The health condition of pet-owners was found to be much better. They had less risk of cardiovascular disorders, lower blood pressure and lower blood cholesterol levels. In another recent study pet-owners were found to receive fewer prescribed medications for cardiovascular problems and to be generally in much better shape.

Results indicating the benefits of pet-ownership were also reported in other countries. In 1991 researchers at Cambridge University found that just months after purchasing a cat or dog, the pet-owner suffered less from such common ailments as flu, headache or backache. In another study, pet-owners who suffered from heart attacks improved quicker than those who did not have pets. A follow-up study has shown that only one of a group of 87 dog owners died in the follow-up year (1%), compared with 19 deaths in the non-owners group of 282 people (7%). Since owning a cat or dog reduces the risk of cardiovascular disease, it may help in prolonging your life.

Can music prolong your life?

According to Californian psychologist Dr. Steve Halpern, "having the right music around the house is as important as having the right food and the right vitamins." Soft music is said to decrease elevated blood pressure, help stabilise heart rate and encourage relaxation. Dr. John Kabat-Zinn, Director of the Stress Reduction and Relaxation Unit at the University of Massachusetts Medical Center also recommends music to his patients. He points out that "music takes the mind to another place, reduces the awareness of pain and puts your psyche someplace else for a while, in a place where there is no pain—psychic or physical."

Today, music is being played in some US hospitals to reduce stress after surgery; it also helps to overcome emotional depression. Music can be an effective therapeutic agent because it stimulates the formation by the brain of natural opiates that produce a pleasurable feeling and decrease feelings of pain and discomfort. Although music therapy is not yet widespread, in some medical centers, especially in the USA, it has been used to alleviate arthritic pain and to treat some neuromuscular problems and bone conditions.

We suggest that readers devote some time to listening to music they like because it would make them feel better, particularly after an unpleasant or stressful event.

Is moderate alcohol intake good for you?

A large number of studies point out that light to moderate alcohol drinking—not more than two drinks per day—causes a modest reduction in coronary heart disease. However, even these 'responsible' levels can significantly increase the risk of some cancers. Researchers at Harvard Medical School, for instance, found that alcohol consumption increases the risk of breast cancer. Women who consumed one or more alcohol drinks per day were found to increase their breast cancer risk by 50 percent when compared to non-drinkers. On the other hand, in a study conducted by the US National Cancer Institute, moderate alcohol drinking was associated with an increased breast cancer risk of up to 100 percent.

Alcohol consumption is also linked to cancers of the mouth, throat, larynx and oesophagus. Moderate levels of alcohol intake also increase the risk of liver cirrhosis by up to 83 percent.

Some researchers point out that these increased risks are offset by the reduced rates of heart disease, stroke and gallstones related to the protective effect of light to moderate alcohol consumption. However, as Dr. Ivan Gyarfes, Chief of Cardiovascular Diseases at WHO points out, "It would be irresponsible to advocate moderate alcohol consumption as a means of preventing coronary heart disease." This approach is supported for two reasons: firstly, the risk of moderate drinking becoming heavy drinking; secondly, the link between alcohol consumption above two drinks per day (about 24 g of ethanol), and increased morbidity and mortality from cardiovascular disease. As Dr. Gyarfes explains, "As a strategy for reducing heart disease it would be much better to address the most important risk factors by promoting smoking prevention, healthy nutrition, regular exercise and hypertension control."

In addition, it has been found that even moderate alcohol consumption can adversely affect brain functions. Researchers were able to identify a group of susceptible individuals in whom brain damage occurs even when they are moderate drinkers.

It has been revealed that after heavy bouts of alcohol consumption there is decreased performance on intelligence tests the next day. In fact, alcohol can kill more brain cells than some of the most dangerous hard drugs.

Alcohol is also a potent source of kilojoules, so if you are overweight and a heavy drinker you may reduce your weight by cutting down sharply or giving up alcohol.

Being intoxicated from alcohol and doing something significant at the same time is particularly hazardous to your chances of living a good and long life. In fact, alcohol intake is involved in more than 50 percent of all road accidents and 50 percent of cases involving pedestrians. Alcohol is also a factor in 60 percent of drownings and many serious domestic accidents. Over 70 percent of men who committed break-ins were to some extent influenced by alcohol. It has been estimated that an alcoholic lives 10 years less than an average person.

Many prescribed drugs can augment the hazardous effects of alcohol. Sleeping tablets can slow down the rate at which alcohol is used by the body. A person who drank in the evening and then took sleeping pills may still be over the legal blood alcohol concentration the next morning.

Alcohol, in whatever amount, is most hazardous to the foetus, particularly during the first three months of pregnancy. The most severe type of defect associated with consumption of alcohol by a pregnant mother is known as foetal alcohol syndrome. Children with this syndrome are mentally retarded and half of them have heart problems.

Is caffeine a life shortener?

Coffee, tea and soft drinks such as the popular cola drinks contain caffeine[1]. Consuming large amounts of these drinks can be hazardous to your health. They may cause abnormally rapid heart beat and may increase blood sugar levels by inhibiting the metabolism of glucose. In a recent study, drinking more than five cups of strong coffee per day was associated with up to a 70 percent increased risk of a first non-fatal heart attack. However, drinking less than six cups daily was found not to increase the risk.

In some people even a few sips of strong coffee or other caffeine-containing drinks may augment blood sugar levels and cause heart rate and blood pressure to rise. These effects may be accompanied by nervousness and irritability.

Heavy consumption of coffee was found to increase blood cholesterol levels even in otherwise healthy people. Some researchers suspect that high regular intake of caffeine may be associated with an increased rate of cancer of the kidney, bladder and pancreas.

Caffeine stimulates acid secretion which may be harmful to people who suffer from stomach ulcers. In addition, the increased acid secretion by caffeine blocks the uptake of calcium which may lead to osteoporosis.

---

[1] On average, a cup of coffee contains about 50% more caffeine than a cup of tea. A can of cola drink can contain the caffeine of one cup of coffee.

There were cases of people who had to give up their jobs because of severe headaches. It was later found that the cause of this symptom was excessive coffee drinking; after some initial symptoms of withdrawal the headaches disappeared when they stopped drinking coffee.

How harmful is tobacco?

Tobacco is probably the worst enemy of longevity. Recent research shows that the effects of smoking are worse than originally thought. It has been revealed that 50 percent of smokers who commence in adolescence will die prematurely as a result of smoking. Half of these deaths will occur in middle age.

Millions of people die every year from cancer and heart disease as a result of smoking. Recent studies indicate that smokers are more likely to get Alzheimer's disease than non-smokers.

Smoking increases the ageing process. Carbon monoxide and nicotine absorbed during tobacco smoking speed up the ageing of arteries, which may lead to degenerative diseases of the arteries. As Dr. P. A. Dupont from Flinders University Medical School in Adelaide, explains, "What we are finding is that men in the 40–60 age group have the arteries of 80-year-olds and it is simply because they have ignored the message—quit smoking." Elderly men are losing their limbs because they could not stop smoking. In Adelaide alone, some 200 elderly patients are having limbs amputated each year for this single reason. As a result of their smoking habit, many thousands of patients cannot walk more than 200 yards without experiencing pain in their legs.

Passive smoking is dangerous too. It has been estimated that nearly 50,000 Americans die each year from lung cancer as a result of involuntary smoke exposure. The more people smoke in your vicinity, the greater the risk.

And what about the so-called smokeless tobacco? It is estimated that about 22 million teenagers and college students use snuff or chewing tobacco in the US. In relation to the lung cancer hazard, smokeless tobacco is safer, but in the case of cancers of the mouth, tongue, oesophagus and pharynx, drain cleaner could not be much more abrasive than tobacco. Snuff is said to increase the risk of getting mouth cancer by about 50 times. Lung cancer kills people when they are in their 50s, oral cancer strikes children. As Dr. Engelstrom notes: "There are reports of 16- and 17-year-olds who needed to have their jaws removed because of oral cancer, and that's just after chewing tobacco snuffs for three or four years."

Recent research has proven earlier reports that smoking can cause premature wrinkles. Wrinkling was shown to increase with the duration of smoking. Heavy smokers are about five times more likely to be wrinkled than non-smokers.

Smoking is particularly hazardous in pregnancy. In the US smoking by pregnant women causes about 14,000 prenatal births each year. Since the bloodstream of a mother who smokes has less oxygen available for the developing foetus, this may cause defects of the baby's central nervous system. Smoking during pregnancy may also impair the growth of the infant's lungs; this may contribute to lung problems in later life.

It is estimated that if a person stops smoking by the age of 35, their chances of living until 70 would be the same as for those who have never smoked. Even for smokers between the ages of 65 and 74, it is worth giving up because the relative survival rates are still higher than for those who continue to smoke.

Is marijuana safer than tobacco?

Marijuana (*Cannabis sativa*) is the most popular recreational drug in Western countries after alcohol and tobacco. It is estimated that 20 million Americans are regular users of marijuana.

About 10 percent of Australian 15-year-olds use marijuana on a weekly basis. Most youngsters believe that marijuana is less dangerous than tobacco. This view is erroneous. As the former Australian Medical Association President, Dr. Brendan Nelson states, "Marijuana is more dangerous than tobacco." It is in fact more carcinogenic than tobacco, particularly as a cause of cancers of the throat and jaw. Marijuana smoke contains more cancer-causing substances than cigarette smoke. It is particularly harmful to the lungs because users of marijuana typically inhale the unfiltered smoke deeply and hold it in their lungs for a prolonged period of time.

This drug is also associated with increased risk of mental illnesses such as schizophrenia. Tetrahydrocannabinol, the main active ingredient of marijuana, has been shown in animal studies to reduce efficiency of the immune system, thereby increasing the risk of infections. Marijuana is a particular hazard in pregnancy as it shows toxic effect on the foetus.

Is occasional use of cocaine safe?

As early as the 1970s cocaine was regarded as a relatively harmless drug when used occasionally. Most official sources dealing with hard drugs asserted that cocaine was not an addictive drug, despite the fact that psychological dependence might take place. Nowadays cocaine is described as one of the most hazardous hard drugs. Deaths have been reported from the use of surprisingly low doses of cocaine. Researchers speculate that some people may have an underlying serious heart condition that is triggered by a small dose of cocaine which for others is not lethal.

Cocaine increases the blood pressure and heart rate. Its use has been linked to heart attacks and stroke and it may trigger an attack of angina. Crack, which is sold as a recreational drug, is a form of cocaine so it is also dangerous. There is some evidence that these drugs may directly harm the immune system and reduce our resistance to infection and other diseases.

Can inhalants cause cancer?

Inhalants are volatile solvents which are used in many commercial products such as glues, paints and motor car fuels. They are also found as ingredients in various cleaning liquids and nail-polish removers. When inhaled these solvents produce intoxication with similar effects to alcohol. Inhalants, which are much cheaper than alcohol, are popular among some youths who use them to get a 'high'. It has been estimated that in the United States 13 percent of young people aged 18–25 have used various inhalants as recreational drugs.

Inhalants are extremely dangerous. Prolonged use of inhalants is a life-threatening habit. Inhalants such as benzene are particularly dangerous; they may cause leukaemia. Toluene may cause permanent degeneration of a part of the brain. Also extremely hazardous are the so-called halogenated hydrocarbons such as trichloroethylene. Long-term exposure to such inhalants may cause liver and kidney damage and serious disease of the nervous system. Trichloroethylene is a common ingredient of dry cleaning agents.

Ecstasy — Can it cause brain damage?

In recent years the drug called ecstasy has become a popular recreational drug among young people. In one study, 40 percent of students at a major university in Australia reported at least experimental use of this drug. Ecstasy is among the most dangerous hard drugs. The deaths of two young people have been reported in Australia in 1995 as a result of using this drug.

Ecstasy has a detrimental effect on the nervous system. Studies have revealed that ecstasy causes certain brain cells to lose many of their projections (called axons), which make contact with other cells in the brain. Although damaged brain cells can develop new axons, animal experiments show that these cells regrow abnormally. There is strong scientific evidence that ecstasy users put themselves at risk of irreversible brain damage.

How dangerous are other illegal drugs?

Heroin use constitutes about 80–90% of narcotic abuse in Western countries. The life expectancy of heroin addicts is significantly lower than that of the general population. Furthermore, withdrawal symptoms are horrific while overdose can lead to death.

If a heroin addict buys pure heroin and is not tolerant of the dose, he or she may die in minutes after injecting. In addition, infections from unsterile needles, syringes, and solutions used may cause many serious diseases. Intravenous drug users can pass on AIDS with their shared (unsterilised) needles.

Another drug called 'angel dust' (phencyclidine) has caused many accidental deaths resulting from erratic behaviour brought on by the drug. Its direct effect on the body has led to some fatalities.

Amphetamines are also hazardous. Heavy use can produce brain damage while death can result from overdose.

How stress shortens your life

A number of health problems are related to prolonged stress. Atherosclerosis, palpitations and heart disease are examples of health problems caused by stress which can actually kill you. Stress can also be harmful to your digestive system, causing nervous diarrhoea, ulcers and constipation. You can also suffer from insomnia, migraine, irritability and hypertension. Stress can lead to depression and even mental illness. Stress has also been linked to asthma, allergies, dermatitis and dyspepsia. One can also feel tired and fragile as a result of stress.

According to the journal *Epidemiology* (July 1993), prolonged stress increases the risk of some cancers. Swedish researchers conducted a study which involved 1000 people. The researchers examined their subjects' medical histories and asked about their major life events during the last 10 years. They concluded that serious work-related problems made an individual five times more likely to have colorectal cancer, and among those who were unemployed for more than six months, the cancer risk was doubled. Moving more than 120 miles made a person three times more likely to develop these cancers. Death of the spouse or divorce increased cancer risk by 50 percent.

Adopting a balanced lifestyle can significantly diminish the amount of stress. First of all, one needs to sleep regular hours and sufficiently long. Regular exercise and appropriate nutrition would also help. Frequent holidays will give new energy to face any future stressful situations. Research revealed that people who took holidays for 15 consecutive years live, on average, five years longer than those who did not.

Try to focus on positive aspects and forget the negative by preoccupying yourself during your spare time with something which has no connection with the stressful event. Plan your time well in advance so that you will have more than enough time to deal with threatening situations. Avoid situations in which there is uncertainty, and finally, practice refusing something nicely. Try to believe you can do something about reducing or eliminating stress from a given situation.

An effective strategy is to find a physical outlet for the powerful feelings of tension and frustration involved that will not do harm to others. This can be accomplished by thumping a punch bag or ripping up waste paper. It can also be done by engaging in physically exhausting exercise, such as jogging or cycling or pulling out weeds.

For some people a better way would be a more passive pursuit such as massage, yoga and meditation. Some commonly used 'remedies' for stress such as heavy drinking or using tranquillisers, can be hazardous to your health.

Can a positive attitude prolong life?

It has been observed that, following surgery, some patients of the same age and health condition recover faster than others. For a long time it has been claimed that these patients recover faster simply because they expect to get well soon. Recently it has been discovered that this claim has scientific foundation because a strong expectation of success can change the level of certain hormones which stimulate the healing process. The brain regulates the activity of the immune system and other systems of the body. The 'thinking' part of the brain can send signals to the hypothalamus, which in turn directs the pituitary gland to release various hormones. These hormones control the endocrine system which regulates all important body functions. This explains why we can improve the speed of our recovery from disease and may even enhance our life expectancy just by having a positive attitude.

According to some gerontologists an individual's state of mind is an important factor in maintaining youth. They argue that people who seem to be always young are always busy with the present and always have an optimistic attitude about their future. When the things and people around them change, they accept this as inevitable and do not worry about it. They seem to send an important message—why worry if I have no influence on what is happening?

Can your thoughts kill you?

There is convincing evidence that lack of will to live can significantly shorten your lifespan.

A destitute woman was successfully treated for tuberculosis in a Denver hospital. However, it was soon noticed that the woman had no will to live and kept saying, "I'm going to die." Within two weeks of her discharge from hospital she died, although an autopsy showed no relevant pathology. Researchers at the University of Massachusetts reported several similar cases. A healthy 76-year-old man, for example, declared that he had decided to die, and he did so three days after selling his house. No physiological cause of death was identified.

The killing power of thought has long been known to people in various regions of the world, for example among Australian Aborigines. In one reported case a healthy young man angered his elders by breaking taboo. The tribal elders held a special meeting during which the so-called medicine man pointed a 'magic' bone at the young man, saying that he would die. Soon after the ceremony the young man was unable to stand, and his body seemed to become paralysed. His breathing became difficult and he looked as though he was about to die. When he was admitted to hospital, he was critically ill although there was no trace of any disease. The man survived only because he was attached to an artificial lung. When asked what happened to him, he admitted that he was dying but survived because the artificial lung destroyed the power of the magic bone.

Can laughter help you live longer?

There is some evidence that laughter can prolong life. According to Dr. William F. Frey Jr, Associate Professor of Psychiatry at Stanford University: "By watching shows that make you laugh and avoiding shows full of violence you can clearly add years to your life." According to Dr. Lee Berk, neurologist of Loma Linda University, California, laughter inhibits the release of stress-related hormones. In fact it has been revealed that 10 minutes of laughter a day can improve circulation and lower blood pressure. Laughter also has a profound effect on our immune system by increasing the number of activated T-cells, B-cells and immunoglobulins, thus making us less susceptible to various infectious diseases. In addition, laughter prompts the release from our brain of natural opiate-like substances known as endorphins, thus reducing pain without the use of medication.

A recent study performed at Mannheim University in Germany shows that not only laughter but even smiling can have a beneficial effect on our health. The researchers claim that smiling and expressing cheerfulness activate facial muscles which influence the brain. The German researchers found that even the "simple art of grasping an object between our teeth and effectively faking a smile causes a 'positive smile response' in our brain."

Watching humorous films that cause us to laugh boosts our immune system. In one study, healthy subjects who watched a humorous show on TV for a long time showed a significant increase in interferon-gamma, not only just after viewing but even the next day. Interferons are proteins secreted by certain body cells which, when taken by other cells, increase resistance to viruses. In this way laughter may become a strong weapon against infection.

It is believed that a sense of humour is not an inborn personality trait—our attitudes can be changed.

Dr. Stephen Jewett, a psychiatrist, scrutinised the lives of 79 men and women aged between 87 and 100. All of them had a great sense of humour and laughed a lot. For example, Anna Mary Moses, the famous US painter, when asked on her 100th birthday how to live to be a 100, replied "Laugh a lot. Tell jokes. If you are alone think of jokes. Keep happy. Keep busy. That's how to do it."

Can faith influence your life expectancy?

More than 200 scientific studies have shown that people who believe in God tend to be healthy when compared to non-believers. The most significant effects were observed in blood pressure. As a rule those who regularly attended church had lower blood pressure than non church-goers.

Several studies have revealed that regular church-goers had half the risk of dying from coronary artery disease when compared to those who rarely go to church, once smoking and other risk factors were taken into account.

A 1996 study of 4000 elderly people living at home, conducted by the National Institute of Aging in Carolina, has shown that those who were strong believers and church-goers were much healthier than those who did not participate in church worship and prayed at home.

A 1995 study at Dartmouth-Hitchcock Medical Center showed that the strongest predictor of survival after heart surgery was the degree to which patients believed that God would give them strength to recover from their illness. The non-believers had more than three times the death rate of believers.

It was found that those people who were both religious and had good social support had a 14-fold advantage in recovery over those who were irreligious and isolated.

Recent studies demonstrate that prayer helps in the same biochemical way as a relaxation response, that is, it causes lowering of blood pressure and decreases heart rate.

Can social position affect your life expectancy?

Researchers who studied a large group of people found that there was a correlation between social class and life expectancy. Those who lived a long life belonged to a higher social class during most of their life; this is usually associated with a good financial position. Seventy percent of the long-lived men admitted that they had high living standards, while only 20 percent of the short-lived men were satisfied with their living standard.

Good income usually means a better diet, more leisure time, job satisfaction, and what is quite important, access to the best quality health care. It has been found that such well paid professionals as physicians, architects, lawyers and scientists usually live longer than people in other occupational groups. Farmers are the only non-professionals who have higher than average life expectancy.

The lower lifespan for those in lower status occupations may be due to poor working conditions and occupational illnesses as well as lower job satisfaction. Since low income normally accompanies low occupational status, the income variable may be the key factor here.

The level of education also seems to influence life expectancy. Studies by the Metropolitan Life Insurance Company (USA), for instance, have revealed that the life expectancy of male university graduates was significantly higher than that of the general white male population, and those with honours degrees lived even longer.

Intelligence level also seems to positively influence life expectancy. The higher an individual's IQ, the longer their life expectancy. Gifted children can serve as an example. Investigation of the progress of a group of gifted children who were observed for 35 years has revealed that they had a much longer life expectancy than the population as a whole.

Long-lived women were found to score about 50 percent better on IQ tests that those women who had an average lifespan. It is not known whether higher than average intelligence is directly linked to longevity. It is possible that individuals with higher intelligence simply choose a lifestyle which is more healthy.

How can you prevent accidents?

When 103 US health experts were asked for their advice on the most important things people could do to promote longevity, six of the main tips were safety precautions:

- Wear your seat belt
- Do not drive after drinking
- Drive within the speed limit
- Have a house with a smoke detector
- Do not smoke in bed (if you can't quit)
- Take precautions against home accidents.

Accidents are the fourth leading cause of death in Western countries. They are the number one cause of death of people under 38. In 1984, in the US alone, there were 9 million disabling injuries, including 92,000 fatalities.

However, you can prevent many accidents. Alcohol is involved in more than half of all road accidents. Even two beers may significantly impair driving skills. It is also dangerous to swim when under the influence of alcohol. More than 60 percent of drowning victims had alcohol in their blood.

Alcohol, however, is not the only mood-and-mind altering substance. Tranquillisers such as Valium have also been shown to be factors in many accidents, as have barbiturates which are used as sleeping pills. A study found that among elderly people who had broken their thigh bone in night time falls, 93 percent were barbiturate users.

Marijuana is another factor that leads to accidents. The ability to perform complex tasks may be impaired even 24 hours after smoking pot.

Even if you do not drive under the influence of alcohol and stay within the speed limit you are still in danger from other avoidable factors. If you play your car radio or cassette player at high volume you increase the danger, not only because you block out car horns and other warning sounds, but also because the music can interfere with your ability to concentrate.

Wearing a seat-belt is vital because if you are thrown out of the vehicle, you are 25 times more likely to die. Even at slow speeds you must wear your seat-belt.

A driver without a seat-belt in a head-on crash between two vehicles moving at 46 km/hr hits the windscreen and dashboard with the same impact as a person hitting the ground after falling out of a third-floor window. In fact you should wear your seat-belt even when you go for a short trip near your home. Seventy-five percent of all accidents occur near home and at speeds less than 65 km/hr. Some people are scared of being trapped by their seat-belt in case of fire or submersion after an accident. Safety experts say, however, that you have a better chance of escaping if you are wearing a seat-belt, because the protection it gives you leaves you in a better shape to deal with your situation. Furthermore, to avoid accidents you should stop and rest every two hours when driving. Finally, never get behind the wheel when you are upset or troubled because people in that state get distracted and cannot give their full attention to driving.

After car accidents, falls are the next most common cause of accidental death. For every four people killed on the roads, one dies in a fall. Because of the dangers associated with falls on stairs you are advised to always:

- Keep your stairs clear
- Do not use your stairs as a storage area

- Have a sturdy handrail beside the stairs.

Accidents often occur in or around bath tubs. You should have:

- A grab bar that will withstand your full falling weight (not a towel rack or soap dish)
- A non-slip surface or mat on the bottom of the bath.

Eighty percent of industrial accidents are caused by stress. You can substantially decrease the chances of such accidents by using techniques that reduce stress, such as having pets, meditation, taking holidays, and having hobbies.

Exercise can significantly reduce your chances of having an accident. Exercise prevents the slowing down of reaction time that usually appears with age. In one study researchers compared fit older people with sedentary people of similar age and found that those who exercised had the reaction times of much younger people. Elderly people who did not exercise had the slowed reaction expected of their age group. Regular exercise may also help maintain good balance by providing the agility to avoid a blow or an obstacle.

Overweight people have significantly more accidents than people of average weight. In fact, most serious industrial accidents happen to people who are 15 percent or more overweight. Overweight people also happen to have more car accidents. One of the reasons for this is lack of physical fitness.

Exercise also helps you to cope with stress, another factor behind many accidents. Finally, if your fitness programme includes walking or other weight-bearing exercises, if you have an accident your bones will probably be stronger and better able to heal breaks.

Sun screen lotions — Can they protect you from skin cancer?

According to a recent study by Margaret L. Kripke and her colleagues at the University of Texas, sun screens help protect against mild skin cancer but appear to be unable to stop ultraviolet rays impairing the ability of immune cells to fight melanoma, the deadliest of skin cancers. Thus, the only advice which can be given is to avoid too much sun exposure or perhaps give up altogether the beach lifestyle so popular in Australia.

When you are in the sun, put on a shirt with long sleeves and wear a wide-brimmed hat. Apply a sun screen with a sun protection factor (SPF) of 15+. Sun screens should be applied to clean, dry skin at least 10–15 minutes before going out in the sun. When you swim or if you perspire heavily, use a sun screen that is water proof or water resistant. Re-apply the sun screen every hour. Stay out of the direct sun between 11.00 AM and 3.00 PM.

Try to work or relax in outdoor areas that are shaded by trees or artificial shade which can help protect you from the sun. Australia has the highest incidence of skin cancer in the world. In fact, two out of three Australians have had skin cancer at some time during their life. About 1000 Australians die each year from skin cancer (mainly malignant melanoma). Thus if you want to live longer, be careful in the sun. In fact, according to researchers, sun screens have another side. By preventing the pain and redness of sunburn most people stay longer in the sun, thus increasing the risk of developing deadly melanoma.

Sunglasses — Can they prevent eye cancer?

Just as your skin is vulnerable to the ultraviolet rays from the sun, so are your eyes. People who live in 'sunshine' countries like Australia and all people who have outdoor jobs, even in temperate countries, are vulnerable to cancer of the eye. This can be easily prevented—wear sunglasses or spectacles that have been treated to block out UV light. Surprisingly, not all sunglasses can protect you from eye cancer. Over 40 percent of sunglasses do not filter out the ultraviolet rays. You can ask your optician for UV-filtering lenses for your spectacles that will filter 90–100% of UV rays without a darkening effect.

You can also protect your eyes by wearing sunglasses that meet the Australian standard (AS 1067). This means that such sunglasses meet the guideline for UV filtration set by the Australian National Standards Institute.

If you are selecting ordinary sunglasses and not looking for those that meet the Australian standard, remember that darker glasses allow greater, deeper penetration of ultraviolet light because their denser colour forces the pupil of the eye to open up. You should therefore only select sunglasses which have grey–brown or grey lenses.

Is exercise always good for you?

Exercise is good for you provided you do not overdo it. A 30-year-long study of the health of 17,000 male Harvard alumni aged 25–74, revealed that those individuals who lost some 2000 calories a week through regular exercise, lived on average 2.5 years longer. However, among those men who tended to expend more than 3000 calories per week there was a slight increase in mortality. A study of women by Dr. Steven Blair from the Cooper Institute for Aerobic Research, also shows a slight increase in death rate from all causes among women who are engaged in the heaviest form of exercise.

It has been found in many studies that those adults who are inactive or sedentary are at about twice the risk for coronary heart disease and cancer when compared with physically active individuals. Furthermore, if you exercise you increase blood supply to some regions of your brain and as a result your brain will function better. This conclusion was reached after experiments on rats. It was found that rats who exercised grew more blood vessels to the brain, supplying it with more nutrients and improving its efficiency.

Between the ages of 20 and 70, the lung power of a non-exerciser can decline by 40 percent. Between the ages of 50 and 60, a non-exerciser can lose about 20 percent of muscle strength, 35 percent of leg and back power and, in the case of postmenopausal women, up to 30 percent of bone density.

Regular exercise lowers the three major factors associated with coronary heart disease: high blood pressure, too high a cholesterol level in the blood, and excessive weight. In fact, regular moderate exercise can induce a fall in blood pressure of about 10 percent lasting several hours. With regular exercise the pulse rate becomes slower and strengthening of the heart muscle takes place. Consequently, the heart's work becomes more mechanically efficient. Unfortunately, of the age group considered 'at risk' of coronary heart disease—those aged 30–60—about 90 percent in Australia do not exercise at the required level. An hour of brisk walking each day, at about 120 steps-a-minute pace, will expend the number of calories needed to prolong your life by an average 2.5 years.

If you prefer to ride a bicycle, you will need to spend 40 minutes on this activity if you ride fast. Running would require about 20 minutes of your time daily, while 10 minutes of swimming daily, about one hour of golf or 45 minutes of tennis will achieve the same aim. About 40 minutes of moderate aerobic dancing burns a similar amount of calories.

Walking is better than jogging because the latter is not suitable for every age and has a high injury rate, a negligible factor among walkers. The same can be said of some other activities.

Walking might be a good preventative measure in delaying senility. A four-month programme of brisk walking was undertaken by a group of elderly people at the University of Utah. It was found that the subjects who took active part in this test were better able to correctly match numbers and symbols at the end of the walking program. Exercise seems to have a power to expand 'mental powers' in elderly individuals, by improving the body's ability to transport oxygen to the brain.

Chapter Four

LIFE SHORTENING MEDICATIONS

Aconite

Although aconite (*Aconitum napellus*) is one of the most poisonous plants known, it is still being used as a herbal remedy, especially to relieve rheumatic pain. It was a popular remedy in traditional Chinese medicine, and it is also occasionally recommended by some Chinese naturopaths in Australia.

In 1989, there were two cases of severe poisoning in Perth, Western Australia. A 43-year-old man who drank a concoction of aconite root before going to bed, woke feeling 'numb all over'. Soon he became quite weak, his heartbeat dropped to 30 beats per minute and his blood pressure dropped so much that he finally collapsed. Treated in the Coronary Care Unit, the man's heartbeat returned to normal and he was discharged from hospital. Not so lucky was another man, a 30-year-old male nurse who purchased the aconite herbal remedy from the same naturopath. After he drank his medicine he became seriously ill. He suffered from palpitations and developed numbness in his fingers, hands and feet, lips and tongue. When taken to hospital his condition continued to deteriorate and despite resuscitation attempts, he suffered cardiac arrest and died.

Aconite root is a particularly dangerous poison because there is no specific antidote to aconitine, its poisonous ingredient. In order to prevent further poisonings, this plant and all remedies which may contain aconite have been banned in Australia. Nevertheless, some herbalists may still recommend a herbal remedy containing aconite root and a patient may not be warned as to its possible hazard.

Borage

Borage (*Borago officinalis*) is used both as a herbal remedy and as a salad. The leaves and flowers of this plant are used in the form of a tea or tincture to treat rheumatism and respiratory infections. It was even recommended to stimulate the milk flow in nursing mothers.

All parts of the plant have been found to contain pyrrolizidine alkaloids which are known to be highly toxic to the liver as well as carcinogenic. Since 1994, borage has been classified in Australia as a substance which is prohibited for sale, supply and therapeutic use.

Despite this official ban some recently published books on herbal remedies recommend the use of borage, especially for infants. However, infants are particularly vulnerable to the pyrrolizidine alkaloids this plant contains. Borage leaves are still sold as a vegetable despite the evident health hazard. Some herbalists claim that borage contains such a small amount of alkaloids that they cannot exert any toxicity. They ignore the well-established fact that the toxic alkaloids are cumulative. Although the amount of alkaloids in the daily intake may be negligible when consumed over a long period of time—say, a few months or a year—the alkaloids' toxicity builds up to levels that cause irreversible liver damage.

Bracken

Bracken (*Pteridium aquilinum*) is a common fern found in many regions of the world including Australia. It has been used mainly as a green vegetable and is occasionally used in folk medicine for gastrointestinal complaints. The plant had been regarded as entirely safe but recent studies have revealed that bracken can be hazardous to our health. It has been found that the incident of oesophageal cancer is three times higher among Japanese who use this plant in salad. The higher the consumption of this salad in Japan, the higher the rate of stomach cancer. A similar relationship has been established in Wales.

The cancer-inducing property of bracken has been demonstrated in animal experiments, and the carcinogenic substance was isolated. It is called ptaquiloside. When this substance was given to experimental animals, tumour formation was observed in various organs. Because of such a hazard, the use of bracken as a herbal remedy was prohibited in most Western countries including Australia. Bracken consumption is particularly hazardous during pregnancy, since the foetus can easily be exposed to carcinogens through the mother's circulation and placenta.

However, refraining from consuming bracken does not entirely solve the problem. There are other ways in which people may become exposed to dangerous carcinogens found in this plant. Firstly, one can be exposed by breathing the spores of this plant since the spores also contain carcinogenic substances. This may happen when walking in the areas where bracken grows in abundance. Secondly, one can become exposed to bracken poisoning by drinking water drained from bracken-covered slopes. Thirdly, poisoning may occur as a result of eating vegetables grown in the soil in which bracken was used as a manure. Finally, one may drink milk from cows grazing on bracken-covered fields.

Calamus

The herb sweet flag (*Acorus calamus*) is a source of the essential oil which may be obtained from the rhizomes. Called calamus oil it has been used as a remedy to treat various ailments, especially rheumatism and gout. Both the plant and its oil were regarded as entirely safe until recently when its toxicity was revealed. Beta-asarone, the main ingredient in calamus oil, was found to cause severe liver damage and to initiate tumour growth in experimental animals.

Although no cases of severe poisoning from calamus oil have so far been reported in humans, it had to be banned as a remedy in most Western countries including Australia. Despite this, caution should be exercised because some less-informed naturopaths may recommend calamus oil to their patients. Calamus oil may still be used in aromatherapy in the belief that when used externally, it cannot be harmful. This is not true. In massage, the oil is usually applied to large areas of the skin, so the oil can be absorbed through the skin with some toxic effect. In fact, even a significantly diluted oil preparation used in massage may be hazardous because of its cumulative effects.

Chapparal

Chapparal (*Larrea tridentata*), also called the creosote bush, is native to southern USA and Mexico. As a herbal remedy it is used to treat many diseases, especially leukaemia and various other forms of cancer. Despite the lack of scientific evidence about its anticancer effects, some people still use it in the hope of finding a cancer cure.

The plant was regarded as safe and no side effects had been observed until 1992 when first reports indicated that this remedy was most hazardous. Severe poisoning was observed in some patients who developed jaundice after taking capsules containing chapparal extract for several months. These patients recovered after hospitalisation. But more severe was the case of a 60-year-old US woman who took chapparal for 10 months. This treatment resulted in irreversible liver damage. To save her life a liver transplant had to be performed. In Australia, a 38-year-old man who took a chapparal preparation for several months developed severe inflammation of the liver, but recovered.

In order to prevent further cases of severe poisoning, the use of chapparal was finally banned in Australia.

Chloramphenicol

Chloramphenicol, the first synthetic antibiotic, is among the most effective drugs used to combat severe infections. However, this antibiotic causes serious adverse effects. In a susceptible individual it may cause death. It was estimated that chloramphenicol caused some 10,000 deaths from aplastic anaemia in Japan. Despite warnings to doctors about the risks involved, strict limitations were not introduced for many years; in France and Spain, the drug is even available over the counter. The sale of this antibiotic over the counter has already been banned in the US, England and Australia. In Australia it is a prescription medicine only; it is used to treat severe infections and in cases where other less toxic antibiotics are ineffective.

Coltsfoot

Coltsfoot (*Tussilago farfara*) is a popular medicinal plant mainly used to treat irritating cough, bronchitis and asthma. The leaves and flowers of this plant were common ingredients in many herbal preparations and in a popular herbal tea. It was regarded as entirely safe. However, in 1988 a case in Switzerland revealed the severe toxicity of this plant for the first time. A child was born with such severe liver damage that despite intensive hospital treatment, the child died after five weeks. The culprit was found to be coltsfoot. The child's mother admitted that during her entire pregnancy she drank a herbal preparation containing coltsfoot to relieve some minor symptoms. Although the child's mother did not develop a liver disease, the liver of the foetus was more susceptible to the plant's toxic alkaloids. As with borage, this plant contains pyrrolizidine alkaloids which may cause severe liver damage. The reason the plant's toxicity has been overlooked for such a long time is that symptoms of poisoning occur only after prolonged use of the plant. When the symptoms appear it may often be too late because serious and irreversible liver poisoning may have already occurred.

The use of coltsfoot should also be avoided for another reason. It has been found in animal experiments that coltsfoot induces cancers of various organs. Although such hazards can only be confirmed in animals, the cancer-causing effect may also be suspected in humans. Because of its strong toxicity coltsfoot has been banned as a herbal remedy in Australia and in other countries. Unfortunately, coltsfoot is sometimes still included in books on herbs without mention of its toxicity.

Comfrey

The roots and leaves of comfrey (*Symphytum officinale*) have been used for many centuries to treat stomach ulcers, irritable cough and many other ailments. Until recently, comfrey preparations were regarded as entirely safe since no adverse effects were observed from its use. The toxicity of this popular herbal remedy was first revealed in the 1980s when fatal liver damage in some individuals was traced to the long-term use of comfrey. This plant was found to contain pyrrolizidine alkaloids which are known for their strong toxic effects. As occurs with coltsfoot first symptoms of liver poisoning may occur after a long time. This is also the reason why comfrey toxicity has only been noticed in recent years. Pyrrolizidine alkaloids found in comfrey are also carcinogenic in experimental animals, hence they are potentially carcinogenic in humans. Because of this possibility and the liver damage it may cause, comfrey has been banned in most Western countries including Australia. Only the external use of comfrey in the form of ointments is regarded as safe. Some authors of even recently published books on herbal remedies ignore the plant's toxicity. Some uninformed people, especially among the elderly, may still grow comfrey in their gardens and use it in the form of herbal tea.

Three other medicinal plants also contain pyrrolizidine alkaloids. One of them is heliotrope (*Heliotropium* species) which is occasionally used to treat skin disease, especially psoriasis. A number of deaths have been reported in India and

Hong Kong. The two remaining herbs are the common ragwort (*Senecio jacobaea*) used for treating rheumatism and respiratory ailments, and butterbur (*Petasites hybridus*) used for treating bronchitis, cough and asthma. The use of these herbs has been banned in Australia, but some people may ignore this advice or be unaware of the risks involved.

Pokeweed

The herbal tea from the roots of the pokeweed (*Phytolacca decandra*), a plant native to North America, was a popular anti-rheumatic remedy in the US. The use of this plant has been banned in the United States because it caused severe poisoning. In the USA it accounted for more than 100 reported cases of poisoning. Pokeweed is still legal in Australia where it is mainly used in the form of ointment, especially to treat cracked nipples and sinusitis. However, even external use of pokeweed preparations is not safe.

The toxic substances in pokeweed can be absorbed through skin abrasions and this may lead to serious blood poisoning. In fact, this plant is so hazardous that those who handle it during collection without gloves are at risk. The plant is especially hazardous to children, and blood abnormalities have been detected just by touching the fresh plant. The highly poisonous substances are called phytolacca toxins, and they are known to induce tumours in experimental animals because of their mitogenic effects. Thus, this plant should not be used as a herbal remedy in any form.

Sassafras

Until recently, the bark of sassafras (*Sassafras albidum*) has been used in the treatment of various ailments. It was mainly used as a general tonic in the form of herbal tea. It was also used in the treatment of rheumatic conditions, as well as a cough medicine. The pure volatile oil (sassafras oil) isolated from this plant was a popular remedy used to treat rheumatic pains, gout, and certain skin conditions such as psoriasis and eczema. Both the oil and the bark preparations were regarded as entirely safe.

It has been found recently that safrole, the main ingredient of the oil which occurs in the bark, is highly toxic and may cause liver damage. Even external use of the pure oil in the form of massage is not safe, because the toxic ingredient can be easily absorbed through the skin and exert its toxic effect.

Animal tests have also shown that safrole as well as the oil of sassafras induces tumours of the liver and other organs. Although no cases directly related to the use of sassafras in humans has so far been reported, because of the proven carcinogenic effects in animals this plant must be considered hazardous and potentially carcinogenic in humans.

Both the sassafras oil and the bark have already been banned as a herbal remedy in Western countries including Australia. Nevertheless, some recently published books available in Australia present this plant as a safe herbal remedy. Some naturopaths may not be aware of the new regulations and may recommend this plant for medicinal use.

Slimming remedies

In 1990 a number of Belgian clinics which specialised in slimming therapy decided to improve the medication used by adding to its formula some Oriental natural products. They chose two herbal remedies, namely *Stephania tetrandra* and *Magnolia officinalis* which were imported from China. It was assumed that these two plants, traditionally used in Chinese medicine, would improve their slimming therapies by preventing abdominal distension and eliminating water retention.

Unfortunately, after just a few months of the treatment with the 'improved' medication some women began to complain that they had some kidney problems. It was soon revealed that these women suffered from severe impairment of kidney function, and in some cases kidney damage was diagnosed. Such adverse effects of the new medication were observed after five months' use. A total of 48 women were identified in Belgium with various degrees of kidney failure, and 18 of the patients required renal replacement therapy.

Once the toxicity of the new medication had been revealed these herbs were immediately excluded from the slimming medication.

Another medicinal plant which became a popular slimming remedy was germander (*Teucrium chamaedris*). In recent years this plant was commonly used in France. French medical scientists became so enthusiastic about the benefit of this remedy that by 1986 it had been officially approved for weight reduction.

Germander, which was regarded as an entirely safe remedy, was soon found to have serious side effects. Between 1986 and 1992 some 30 cases of severe liver poisoning were observed in some patients who took it for a long period of time. There was even one fatal case reported in France in 1992. A 68-year-old woman who took germander to lose weight became seriously ill. She was brought to a local hospital where irreversible liver damage was diagnosed. And this happened after using the plant for just six weeks. Because of her age liver transplant could not be recommended and the woman died.

The plant has been thoroughly investigated and a diterpene was found to be the toxic plant ingredient. The use of this highly hazardous remedy was officially banned in France in 1993. Since germander was traditionally regarded as entirely safe it may still be recommended by some naturopaths who are not aware of its toxicity.

Chapter Five

OTHER LIFE SHORTENERS

Air pollution

In some regions air pollution is an important factor which can be detrimental to our health and which may limit our lifespan. In fact pollution may be a direct cause of premature death. A US Congressional Report points out that in 1980 about 50,000 people died prematurely in North America alone as a result of inhaling toxic substances from polluted air. According to some estimates, up to 25,000 cancer deaths per year in the US have been or are caused by polluted air. Scientists argue that if the air pollution level could be reduced by half, such common diseases as bronchitis could be reduced by 50 percent and coronary heart disease by 15 percent.

The most common pollutant in our cities is carbon monoxide which is produced in large amounts by motor vehicles. Carbon monoxide interferes with the capacity of blood to carry and supply oxygen. It has been estimated that almost 20 percent of Washington's commuters who spend 6–10 hours per week travelling into the city and back, are exposed to levels of carbon monoxide exceeding the National Air Standard.

Since the 1940s tetraethyl lead has been added to petrol and consequently large quantities of poisonous lead have been dispersed as dust into the air. In 1980 some 1000 tonnes of toxic lead dust from vehicle exhausts were deposited over Sydney alone. Lead is extremely toxic. It causes injury to bone marrow and kidneys. It may also cause serious injury to the nervous system including the brain.

Another substance which may occur in polluted air is ozone. Although the ozone layer found in the upper atmosphere is beneficial as it protects us from dangerous types of solar radiation, ozone near the ground is hazardous to our health. It is formed at lower levels by reactions between oxygen and industrial pollutants in the presence of sunlight. The main precursors of ozone are hydrocarbons and nitrogen oxide, both emitted from car exhausts. More than half of the people in the US are exposed to ozone levels higher than the concentration regarded as safe. Ozone pollution may cause inflammation of the lungs. It may also cause impairment of the immune system. Most hazardous, however, is the ozone cancer-causing effect. Studies have shown that persistent exposure to even low levels of ozone in the air increases the risk of developing lung cancer. In fact, if you choose to live most of your life in a significantly less polluted rural environment, you may add about four years to your life expectancy; if you choose an urban environment, you may shorten your life by two years.

Aluminium

Some researchers argue that aluminium may play a role in Alzheimer's disease and in certain other neurological diseases. Aluminium is found in some drinking water, in some antacid medicines, and it may also be leached from cooking utensils made from aluminium.

A number of studies tend to support the view that aluminium intake may be harmful. Sohler and his colleagues found in their studies that in individuals suffering memory loss the blood level of aluminium was 39.4 parts per billion while in those without memory loss it was 31.3 parts per billion.

The three regions of the world which have the highest aluminium level in their soil also have a high incidence of a motor neurone disorder called amyotrophic lateral sclerosis (ALS) and also Parkinsonism and Parkinson's dementia. These regions also have a low level of magnesium and calcium. Deficiency of magnesium and calcium seems to increase intestinal absorption of aluminium, and its deposition in the central nervous system.

Significant amounts of aluminium were found to accumulate in the brain of the victims of Alzheimer's disease. A British study has revealed that the occurrence of Alzheimer's disease is 1.5 times higher in districts where the aluminium levels in drinking water exceeded 0.11 parts per million, compared with the districts where the level was less than 0.01 parts per million.

People with Alzheimer's disease have a significant decrease in the activity of an enzyme in the brain called choline acetyl transferase. Scientists have shown that aluminium inhibits transport of this enzyme in red blood cells. In addition, aluminium has been found to reduce nerve tissue choline acetyl transferase activity.

It has not been proven that aluminium actually plays a role in these diseases. Nevertheless, to be on the safe side we should try to avoid aluminium intake.

The following precautions should be taken. First, check if aluminium is added to your water supply. If so, we suggest installation of a water purifier or the purchase of water from another source for drinking and cooking.

Buying drinks in aluminium cans should be avoided. Replace your aluminium cooking utensils with stainless steel or use glass cookware. Avoid eating foods which use aluminium in processing or as additives. You can examine additive codes on the packages of food products.

Because aluminium salts are widely used in medical preparations, try to choose aluminium-free alternatives in your pharmacy. Finally, it is a good idea to try to avoid or at least limit the use of the deodorants and antiperspirants which contain aluminium chloride.

Antibiotics in meat

In the US about half of the antibiotics manufactured are used not to treat people, but in the production of farm animals such as cattle, pigs and poultry. They are usually not given to treat infections but to accelerate animal growth and weight. The antibiotics which are given to domestic animals are usually the same as those prescribed for humans. This practice, however, may have a significant effect on human health. As a result of extensive intake of antibiotics by domestic animals the product we obtain from them is loaded with antibiotics. Consequently, when we eat meat, eggs or milk products we may gradually accumulate some antibiotics in our body, and, more importantly, we may develop resistance to bacteria in the same way that we would if we failed to take the full prescribed dosage. By ingesting antibiotics in small portions when we consume meat or other animal products, we give bacteria enough time to either develop resistance to an antibiotic or to develop mutant forms. In any case, the result is such that in the future, the antibiotic in question will not be able to control a similar infection in our system.

Consequently, when a usually effective antibiotic is prescribed to treat a life-threatening disease such as pneumonia, it becomes useless. It has been found in recent years that some people develop an immunity to all known antibiotics, and cases of death occurred because antibiotics were ineffective and the infectious disease could not be cured. According to reports by the Australian Consumer Association, there is a widespread and often illegal use of antibiotics in farm animals. In fact, residues of tetracycline significantly above the permitted levels were detected in 5 of 14 meat samples. This is another reason why it is better to avoid consumption of meat or at least reduce your meat intake.

Artificial sweeteners

Several synthetic substances have been used as sweeteners in Australia. These include cyclamates, aspartame and saccharin.

Both cyclamates and saccharin are not metabolised in the body so their consumption does not add calories and they are very popular among weight-watchers.

Cylamates are sixty times sweeter than sugar and are often used in combination with saccharin or when a heated product requires sweetening. In Australia cyclamates are among the most common artificial sweeteners of diet soft drinks. Cyclamates are also popular sweeteners of various low joule foods, especially canned fruit products and jams.

Research has shown that when cyclamates are fed to experimental animals they can cause bladder cancer. However, the doses which are applied to induce tumour growth in animals are extremely high when compared with the small amounts used in sweetened food products. So, it is assumed that the potential carcinogenic hazard in humans is remote. Nevertheless, because such a hazard cannot be ruled out it is best to avoid their use.

Saccharin, another popular artificial sweetener, is 300 times sweeter than sugar. Some studies have identified a link between saccharin use and the rate of bladder cancer. The Committee on Toxicology in the UK accepted as proven fact that saccharin causes cancer in experimental animals, but did not ban the sweetener because of lack of clear evidence that it may be carcinogenic in humans. The safety of saccharin still remains a controversial issue. Greece, France and Canada banned saccharin in foods and drinks but allowed it to be sold in the form of tablets for diabetics. In the US all products containing saccharin have labels indicating the potential adverse effects. In Australia saccharin is still a popular artificial sweetener used in various diet drinks, canned foods, baked foods, jams and desserts.

The use of aspartame was approved as a sweetening agent in 1981 and, being 200 times sweeter than sugar, it became a popular sweetener. Aspartame is metabolised, and for that reason the increase in one's caloric intake is negligible. Some studies have found that high doses of some sweeteners can possibly cause tumour growth in experimental animals.

Aspartame is hazardous to individuals who suffer from a rare genetic deficiency called phenyloketonuria.

Blue-green algae

High levels of toxic blue-green algae are sometimes found in reservoirs, rivers or lakes supplying water for human consumption. Algae-affected water is responsible for thousands of sheep and cattle deaths in Australia.

There are no recorded human deaths but contamination with blue-green algae can cause serious illnesses in humans. The affected water may cause diarrhoea, vomiting, asthma and liver complications. According to Professor Ian Falconer, a biochemist in the Department of Experimental and Clinical Pharmacology at the University of Adelaide, peptide toxins secreted by the blue-green algae can cause severe respiratory problems, stomach inflammation and serious liver disease. The primary concern, however, is the possible danger of inducing cancer in humans. Blue-green algae are believed to be responsible for stomach and bowel cancer. In Brazil and China algae-contaminated water caused liver damage. Humans can be negatively affected by blue-green algae not only as a result of drinking the contaminated water. When you bathe, shower or come into contact with the water for any other reason it can cause sore throat, skin irritation, itchiness, asthma and hay fever, rashes and other symptoms.

Therefore, we advise readers to find out whether their drinking water is threatened by blue-green algae and, if so or when in doubt, to try to use other sources of drinking water such as bottled spring water. You are also advised to use rubber gloves when washing dishes and clothes in contaminated water. You should hose down filter pads in evaporative coolers once a week. Remember, rain water tanks must be sealed to exclude light, otherwise hazardous algae can grow in them.

Cadmium

Cadmium is a cumulative poison. It can disrupt a number of important enzymes essential to maintaining human health. An impairment of renal function and even kidney damage is associated with increased cadmium intake. Some researchers speculate that the increased incidence of diabetes in Western countries may at least be partly explained by increased cadmium intake. Cadmium was also found to suppress testicular function and has been linked to an increased incidence of prostate cancer.

Experiments have revealed that mice and rats fed a cadmium-free diet lived longer than the animals fed food containing traces of cadmium. High intake of cadmium has also been linked to heart disease.

It is now a common practice in Western countries to use cadmium-containing superphosphate-type fertilisers; consequently, many of our food products, including meat, have unacceptable levels of toxic cadmium. A food survey conducted for the National Health and Medical Research Council of Australia in 1988 revealed the following: 41 percent of potato samples and 28 percent of carrot samples had cadmium levels above the maximum permissible concentration. Twenty-four percent of tested wheat grain samples also exceeded the maximum permissible concentration of cadmium. Another survey revealed that 21 percent of sheep's kidneys contained unacceptable levels of cadmium.

Cadmium pollutes our environment not only because of the use of certain fertilisers. Cadmium is found in zinc ores (0.3%) and is released into the atmosphere during the smelting process. It was estimated that 2300 tonnes of cadmium are released into the air annually over the United States. Cadmium can also be released from burning waste such as plastics, steel scraps and car exhausts. An important source of cadmium in the air we breathe is cigarette smoke. It has been found that tobacco smokers had in their body twice the cadmium levels of non-smokers.

Colouring agents

Over 40 colouring agents are added to various foods in Australia and 26 of those are synthetic substances. These manufactured colouring agents are obtained from coal tar and all have adverse effects. They may provoke severe allergic reactions, even causing asthma in sensitive individuals. Reaction to these dyes may lead to such symptoms as runny nose and eyes, and blurred vision. People sensitive to aspirin and other salicylates are most vulnerable. Because colouring agents added to food are obtained from coal tar they are all suspected of being carcinogenic to humans.

Among the most commonly used synthetic colouring agents is amaranth, also known as Red No. 2. It is added not only to various foods but also to some medicines. As early as the 1960s it had been demonstrated in animal studies that amaranth may cause birth defects and even lead to foetal deaths. Consequently, in 1976 this colouring agent was banned as a food additive in the US, Japan, Norway, Finland, Austria and Greece, but it is still permitted in Australia.

Another hazardous colouring agent (Code No. 102) is tartrazine which is among the most common yellow colouring substances used in food products in Australia. Almost any food product coloured yellow or orange contains some amount of tartrazine. This colouring agent, even if used in a minute concentration, may cause severe asthma attacks in sensitive individuals, although such cases are rare. Some countries, (eg Finland and Norway), have already banned this substance as a food colouring agent.

Electromagnetic radiation

Millions of people may face an increased risk of contracting cancer and degenerative disease because they are exposed to dangerous levels of electromagnetic radiation from power lines and electric appliances. This conclusion is found in a leaked report written by the US government's radiation advisers for the National Council on Radiation Protection. In the report it is argued that safety limits for exposure to electromagnetic fields (EMFs) should become 5000 times lower than the current internationally recommended limits. The report is a draft completed over a period of nine years by a committee of 11 leading American experts in electromagnetic fields. It is the most comprehensive study ever undertaken on the health effects of EMFs.

According to the Committee Chairman Ross Adey, "a powerful body of impressive evidence now exists which suggests that very low exposure to EMFs have long-term harmful effects." Animal studies have shown that the pineal gland is sensitive to weak EMFs and exposure to such EMFs can lead to a decreased production of melatonin by the pineal gland. Decreased production of melatonin has been associated with malignant growths. Recent research has shown that people with Alzheimer's disease tend to have abnormally low levels of melatonin, which suggests that this may be a factor contributing to the disease.

Many studies have revealed that children living near power lines have a higher risk of developing leukaemia. On the other hand adults exposed daily to EMFs at work are at greater risk of developing brain cancer and leukaemia.

It has been also shown that low EMFs exposure could help tumours to grow or cause chemical or genetic damage to cells. Other studies show that EMFs effect the reproductive and immune system. Further studies are needed to clarify the situation. Nevertheless, the report recommends a safety limit of 0.2 microteslas. This recommendation is hard to put into practice because stronger fields are common close to household appliances and electricity pylons. The report says that power lines must be kept away from kindergartens, schools and houses. For existing houses the report advises that radiation be kept "as low as possible" and recommends phasing in the new limit over the next 10 years.

Exposures 30 cm from many household appliances can exceed 0.2 microteslas, often quite significantly. For example, a person standing 30 cm from a vacuum cleaner or electric drill can be exposed to anywhere between 2 and 20 microteslas. Exposure immediately beneath a 400 kV line is about 40 microteslas.

The above views are shared by Sweden's government advisers who demand that new houses should not be exposed to more than 0.2 microteslas.

The British National Radiological Protection Board declined to comment on the leaked report It continues to assert, along with the British electricity industry, that there is no established health risk from low electromagnetic fields. However, Robert McGaughy, a leading expert at the British Environmental Protection Agency, asserts that the agency review of EMFs and the risk of cancer, to be published in 1997, reaches similar conclusions to those in the leaked report.

Thus, we recommend that you do not choose to live next to or in the vicinity of electric power lines, and limit your daily use of household electrical appliances to a minimum.

Fluorescent light

In 1978, a study in the US revealed that women who worked in rooms with fluorescent light had twice the risk of developing malignant melanoma (a type of skin cancer), than women exposed to ordinary types of lighting. The longer the exposure to fluorescent lighting, the greater was the risk.

A study conducted in the US in 1983 has also shown a near double risk of developing malignant melanoma after exposure to fluorescent light at work or at home. Two UK studies have also found a link between exposure to this form of lighting and melanoma (1986 and 1988).

Finally, a Canadian study of 1992 appears to show an increased risk of melanoma associated with exposure to domestic fluorescent lighting. In addition, animal experiments show that fluorescent lighting has mutagenic capability.

Although some previous studies have not shown this melanoma link, the Canadian researchers—on the basis of their results, previous epidemiologic studies, and animal and clinical evidence—maintain that fluorescent lighting is a potential risk factor for humans. Thus, it is better to remain on the safe side and avoid this form of lighting.

Hazardous apple juices

In 1993, the Food and Drug Administration (FDA) in the US conducted a survey of the safety of apple juices found on the market. It was revealed that about 25 percent of fresh apple juices and frozen apple concentrates had higher than permitted levels of the natural toxin patulin. This substance is only found in rotten apples as it is a product of moulds: it would not occur in fresh healthy apples. It was obvious that the tested juices were obtained not from fresh applies, but from much cheaper mouldy apples.

Patulin is a toxic substance and when tested in experimental animals it shows strong immunosuppressive action and is therefore hazardous to our health. In addition, patulin has an effect which resembles that of antibiotics. This causes a problem. Drinking apple juice contaminated with patulin may, over a longer period of time, lead to resistance of the body to certain types of prescribed antibiotics, thus making certain antibiotic treatments ineffective. An investigation is now being carried out to determine other possible risks to our health associated with apple juices containing patulin. It is thus better to avoid an apple juice where there is a suspicion it may be prepared from mouldy apples.

Iron

According to a study published in the *New England Medical Journal* (1988), excessive intake of iron can augment the long-term risk of all types of cancer. It was found that men with high levels of iron in their bodies had up to a 40 percent increase in cancer risk.

Some studies have also linked excessive iron intake to the increased risk of developing coronary heart disease.

Researchers in Finland established that a group of men with high iron intake were more likely to develop coronary heart disease, and that those with high concentrations of iron in their blood were twice as likely to suffer from heart attack.

Too much iron can upset the balance of zinc and copper, leading to constipation. Nevertheless, some iron is absolutely necessary for maintaining good health. Severe iron deficiency has been linked to anaemia and such symptoms as fatigue, irritability and memory disturbance. About 20 percent of Australians take unnecessary iron supplements, thus augmenting their iron intake to dangerous levels, while another 20 percent have an iron deficiency.

Meat and cancer

Another reason for avoiding meat is that it is often preserved with nitrates and nitrites. Examples of such foods include most hams, hot dogs and bacon. Nitrates and nitrites interact with substances called amines in the gastrointestinal tract to form nitrosamines—cancer-causing agents in the stomach and oesophagus. For instance, if you eat a 100 g portion of nitrite-preserved bacon, your body could be absorbing the same amount of hazardous nitrosamines as if you had smoked a pack of cigarettes.

One could point out here that fresh vegetables may also contain nitrates and nitrites. However, most vegetables also contain sufficient vitamin C which has been found to inhibit the formation of nitrosamines.

Tomatoes, carrots and pineapples contain chlorogenic and p-coumaric acids which also suppress the cancer-causing effects of nitrosamines.

Grilled and fried meats are known to promote the formation of the heterocyclic amines which can cause cancer. Recent studies indicate that such meats are not only hazardous when ingested. The vapours emitted during the meat-grilling process contain amines that are hazardous if inhaled. In this way, those who do not consume grilled meat but simply prepare it, may be exposed to its carcinogenic effects. However, the quantity of toxic amines found in 1 gram of grilled or fried meat is about three times more carcinogenic than the amount of these substances found in the fumes emitted by this amount of meat. The charcoal-barbecued meat or fish so popular in Australia cannot be regarded as safe as it is potentially carcinogenic. In 1975, Dr. Raymond J. Shamberger of the Biochemistry Department of the Cleveland Foundation (USA), found that beef contains a strong carcinogenic substance called malonaldehyde. This substance starts to form in beef almost immediately after the animal is slaughtered. Half of the laboratory animals given food containing malonaldehyde developed tumours in three weeks. According to Dr. Shamberger, "we can suspect a similar effect on the human digestive tract when malonaldehyde is carried to it in foods." The carcinogenic effect of the malonaldehyde has so far not been investigated in humans.

Mercury fillings

There is a growing controversy even among specialists about the safety of mercury amalgam fillings. According to the South Australian branch of the Dental Association, "Dental amalgam is a safe, cost-effective material. No grounds exist for recommending discontinuance due to toxicity." The opponents of mercury amalgam point out that, according to the report of the World Health Organisation, no amount of exposure to mercury vapour can be regarded as totally harmless. In fact, some studies have shown that consuming hot food or drink can cause the release of considerable amounts of toxic mercury vapour from dental amalgams.

Some countries have already decided to ban mercury fillings. In Sweden they will be banned by 1997. Austria plans to ban mercury fillings by the year 2000. The use of mercury fillings has already been banned in Germany, and in Japan they have not been used in more than decade. In California dentists who use mercury amalgam must display a warning to their patients about its potential health hazard.

So far it cannot be comprehensively proved than mercury fillings are harmful; neither can we say that they are harmless. To be on the safe side we recommend that you avoid mercury fillings.

Noise

Many studies show that workers exposed to noise at work equivalent to about 90 dB or above have a higher incidence of circulatory disorders than other workers. In 1995, for instance, researchers at La Sapieza University in Rome found that hypertension was more common in Italian men exposed to levels of noise of around 90 dB at work.

Several studies have also linked long-term exposure to traffic noise with increases in blood pressure. In 1995, for example, researchers at the Slovak Academy of Sciences in Bratislava discovered that children attending kindergartens near busy roads (traffic noise no greater than 60 dB), had high blood pressure (*Journal of Hypertension*).

Living near busy airports was also found to cause serious health problems. In fact, the purchase of drugs to treat cardiovascular disease was closely linked to the number of noisy aircraft overflights at night.

Many studies have revealed that noise pollution considerably shortens the life of experimental animals. Rabbits that were exposed to 120 dB noise levels for only 10 weeks developed high blood cholesterol levels and their arteries had atherosclerotic changes.

Researchers point out that the risk of cardiovascular disease increases with the intensity and period of exposure to excessive noise (*International Journal of Angiology*, 1995).

Peanuts

Peanuts and peanut butter can be hazardous to your health because they can be contaminated with toxic substances called aflatoxins. They are produced by certain moulds which may attack peanuts during harvest or storage. Aflatoxins are stable substances so even roasting does not destroy them. They are among the most potent carcinogenic agents, capable of inducing tumours in experimental animals. A link between aflatoxins-contaminated food and liver cancer in humans was suspected long ago and is now confirmed by epidemiological studies. In 1983, Leonard Stoloff carried out a study in various parts of the US on the incidence of liver cancer. He found that there was a 10 percent higher rate of cancer in the areas with high intake of aflatoxins-contaminated food products. A high incidence of liver cancer was also reported from some regions of Africa and Asia characterised by high consumption of peanuts contaminated by aflatoxins.

Although aflatoxins occur mainly in peanuts, they may also be found in other nuts, maize and grains. If a food that contains high amounts of aflatoxins is fed to domestic animals, meat, eggs and even milk may become contaminated with aflatoxins. In this situation it is essential to have proper quality control so that products which contain a high level of aflatoxins are not consumed.

Health authorities allow only minute amounts of aflatoxins in food products. If the level is less than 15 parts per million, the products are regarded as harmless. If the concentration of aflatoxins is higher the product is considered unfit for human consumption. Monitoring this law is not easy and to be on the safe side one should choose only freshly dried peanuts. If they taste somewhat mouldy, it is better not to eat them. Avoid buying peanuts and other food products from places where quality control may be lacking or inadequate.

Pesticides

It has been estimated that about 60 pesticides used in the US are known, or believed to be, carcinogenic; 'believed' means that there is evidence of carcinogenic effect, although contradictory evidence may also exist. Hundreds of other chemicals used in pesticides are still unknown to us; that is, adequate safety testing has not yet been completed.

Most governments allow these hazardous chemicals to be used because it is believed that associated financial benefits outweigh the health risks. One such dubious pesticide is alar. It has been used for about three decades on a variety of agricultural products but mostly on apples. Alar regulates the growth of fruits so that they do not fall from the tree until they are fully ripe. Alar penetrates the fibre of the plant and so it cannot be removed from apples by simple washing. Since the mid-1970s there has been evidence that it may have carcinogenic effects in experimental animals.

Alar residues turn up in a variety of processed apple products, including baby foods. In 1985 the Environmental Protection Agency in the US proposed a ban on the use of alar when there is a potential risk to infants and children—the main consumers of apple products. However, the agency also stated that there is still insufficient evidence, or that the existing evidence of cancer risk is inconclusive, so it did not prohibit the use of alar. Instead of a total ban, the only limitation the agency placed on its use was that the acceptable amount to be used in crops was reduced by 50 percent. Variations of the alar story can be told about many other hazardous pesticides which may be found in our food products.

Few people in Australia realise that many imported foods are treated with pesticides which have been banned in their own country. In fact the US exports some pesticides when these have been banned in the US. In 1980, for example, 25 percent of US pesticide exports consisted of products banned in the US. Some of these pesticides, harmful to health, returned to American consumers in the food imported to the US so there is a so-called 'circle of poison'.

It is assumed that daminozide, maneb, and mancozeb, three pesticides found in imported food products, caused an extra 123,000 cancer cases in the US. It is estimated that in the 1980s some 6000 pre-school children in the US developed cancer solely due to their exposure to pesticide residues from just eight hazardous pesticides found in vegetables and fruit.

A recent survey of American supermarkets revealed the following: 44 percent of 71 vegetable and fruit samples contained residues of 19 different pesticides, and of those, seven are known or believed to be carcinogens. Three of these pesticides—Aldrin, Endrin and DDT—were forbidden in the 1970s.

Dr. Elizabeth Weisburger of the US National Cancer Institute the advises Americans to select a diverse range of vegetables and fruits in order to avoid an overwhelming dose of any one pesticide. In her view, people in Western countries should try to avoid imported fruits as they generally have a higher level of pesticide residue than those grown locally. When buying fruits, it is better to choose less perfect looking ones because they are probably less intensively treated with pesticides. As Dr. Karim Ahmed, Senior Scientist of the Natural Resources Defense in New York advises: "I think, waxed products should never be bought by anyone… It's not clear that paraffin wax isn't carcinogenic itself. And many of the non water soluble products are retained in the wax!"

The simplest way to remove excess pesticides from fruit and vegetables is to peel and wash them; this, however, does not work for all pesticides as some enter the fruit or vegetable itself. Washing with water removes some water-soluble pesticides. Fruit and vegetables should be rinsed thoroughly. This can be more effective if you first bathe the vegetables in water, with a little mild liquid detergent added. The detergent will remove some non water-soluble pesticides. The best solution would be to avoid fruit and vegetables grown with the use of pesticides and consume only those which are organically grown.

Chapter Six

LIFE PROLONGING THERAPIES

Aspirin

Every year some 20,000 Australians die from heart attack, and coronary heart disease is one of the most serious obstacles to achieving longevity. Aspirin might help to reduce this hazard. Studies conducted at Harvard University in the late 1980s confirmed the beneficial effects of this commonly used drug. Half of the 22,071 healthy male doctors who participated in the study took aspirin every other day while the rest took placeboes. Both groups were monitored for five years. Among the participants who took aspirin there were 44 percent fewer cases of heart attack.

There is a scientific explanation for this preventative effect. Aspirin prevents formation of dangerous blood clots, and in this way, when taken regularly as a blood thinner, it becomes an excellent preventative measure against heart attack. Anyone who has a sudden chest pain spreading to the neck or shoulders, or experiences shortness of breath, should immediately take an aspirin tablet because it might be a life saver even during a heart attack.

The National Heart Foundation of Australia advises people, especially the elderly with atherosclerosis and high blood cholesterol levels, to regularly take a small dose of aspirin as a preventative measure.

Studies have shown that regular taking of aspirin may also help to prevent stroke which is caused by a blood clot. In people who have already had a minor stroke aspirin can reduce the risk of a second stroke by nearly 25 percent.

There is also growing evidence that long-term use of aspirin may reduce the risk of certain cancers. The Nurses Health Study reported in the *New England Journal of Medicine* (1995) that women who regularly used aspirin for 10 or more years had a substantial reduction in their risk of colorectal cancer.

In a few individuals even small doses of aspirin may cause adverse effects. Some people are very sensitive to aspirin, especially allergic people, and in such individuals even a small dose of aspirin may trigger a serious and even life-threatening asthma attack. This is why those who intend to regularly use aspirin as a preventative medicine should always contact their doctor first.

Cellular therapy

One of the techniques claimed to slow the ageing process is so-called cellular therapy. It involves intramuscular injection of live cells obtained from the foetuses of sheep. Dr. Paul Niehans from Switzerland, who invented the procedure, believed that the human body would absorb the fresh cells from the unborn lamb and as a result would revitalise itself. He was aware that normally the body rejects 'foreign' cells but he claimed that it does not reject the fresh cells of the unborn lamb. This may be partly true because at the foetal stage cells do not have such characteristic signals by which the body can recognise their foreignness. Nevertheless, most scientists believe that the introduced cells must be destroyed in some way, perhaps slowly.

Niehans used his therapy not only for rejuvenating elderly people but also for treating various diseases. He injected fresh cells obtained from different organs of animal foetuses, depending upon the diseased organ to be cured. For an ailing heart, for example, he would inject the cells of a young sheep heart. The treatment of male impotence involved injecting the cells from the sex glands of the animal. To rejuvenate individuals, he used not only cells from sex glands but also from other organs, injecting them at different times.

His first successful treatment was given to a woman who was critically ill after an unsuccessful thyroid gland operation. Niehans decided to inject her with live cells from the animals' thyroid glands, and this treatment is said to have saved the woman's life. This was in fact the beginning of his career. Niehans' therapy was so expensive however, that only the rich and famous could afford to be his patients. Adenauer, Churchill, Eisenhower and Picasso were among his patients. Niehans was even invited to the Vatican to treat the critically ill Pope Pius XII who had cancer. The Pope believed that it was the Swiss doctor who saved his life because he lived for four years more after the cellular treatment.

Since it is difficult to find a scientifically based explanation of the benefit of cellular therapy and the evidence provided by the proponents of the therapy is anecdotal, mainstream physicians are reluctant to accept Niehans' procedure. Cellular therapy is not allowed in most countries including the US and England. It is still, however, practised legally in Switzerland and Germany as well as in Mexico where there are clinics specialising in cellular therapy.

This therapy is not a safe procedure. As early as 1955 adverse effects resulting from this therapy were revealed in 80 patients in Germany alone. Thirty fatal cases reported in Europe are believed to have been caused by severe allergic reaction to injected animal tissues. Inflammation of the brain and spinal cord were found to be the most hazardous effects of cellular therapy. Because this therapy involves injecting fresh animal tissue there is the hazard of transferring some harmful 'slow viruses' during the treatment, the severe adverse effects of which may occur long after the treatment has been completed.

Cellular therapy is illegal in Australia.

Chelation therapy

Chelation therapy involves a series of intravenous injections of a substance called EDTA (ethylenediaminetetraacetic acid). During this procedure the molecules of the EDTA are supposed to bind (chelate) with any toxic substance found in the bloodstream; the poisonous material, together with the binding substances, is then excreted in the urine.

Chelation treatment can be life-saving in the case of severe poisoning with toxic metals such as lead or copper.

However, this therapy has been used by some physicians as a general treatment for diseases such as coronary heart disease. The proponents of chelation therapy maintain that it can clean the obstructions in the arteries caused by plaques so well that a bypass operation becomes unnecessary. Small wonder that many elderly patients flock to the clinics offering chelation therapy. According to its supporters, the therapy works because it removes all calcium from the atherosclerotic plaques, thus eliminating the source of atherosclerosis. Although this explanation may sound convincing it does not have a scientific basis. This is because artery plaques are mainly composed of cholesterol deposits, while calcium occurs there only in minute quantities. Therefore, even if all calcium was removed by chelation this procedure cannot significantly 'clean' the affected arteries as it is claimed.

To check the supposed beneficial effects of chelation therapy and cardiovascular disease, two double-blind clinical studies have recently been performed in Germany. No improvement in the group of patients treated with chelation could be observed.

Since the beneficial effects of chelation could not be supported by clinical studies, mainstream physicians do not accept the treatment of atherosclerosis by chelation therapy. In fact this therapy may be hazardous. The promise of an easy 'removal' of atherosclerotic buildup in the arteries by chelation may postpone the use of effective treatments currently available.

Some proponents of chelation therapy insist that this treatment can improve sexual vigour in the elderly and that it can prolong life even in those who do not suffer from atherosclerotic disease. These assertions are also without any scientific foundation.

Coenzyme Q_{10}

Coenzyme Q_{10} was identified in 1957. It is an essential part of mitochondria, the cell's energy factory. The amount of this substance in various body cells declines with age. Since ageing is a process which involves rapid degeneration of mitochondria in some cells, it is no wonder that some gerontologists began to speculate that increasing the amount of this coenzyme in the body may slow the ageing process. In animal experiments such a rejuvenating action could be demonstrated. When old mice were given the coenzyme significant improvement of their immune system was observed. This could lead to life extension. Preliminary studies indicate that the coenzyme may help to prevent the formation of atherosclerotic plaque. An antioxidant effect may be involved in this action.

Despite the promising results obtained in experimental animals, there is still no scientific evidence to support the view that the coenzyme Q_{10} can prolong life in humans. Thus, most doctors are sceptical and reluctant to recommend this supplement to their patients.

Deer horn

Among various rejuvenating remedies from the Orient the most popular is the one prepared from the horns of deer. It is an alcoholic extract of the powdered horn, which is produced on a large scale in China and Russia. It is commonly believed that this remedy can not only cure many conditions of the elderly but that it is capable of adding many years to human life. Although the horns of noble spotted deer (*Cervus dyborski*) are considered to be the most potent, they became so rare that other related species are now being used.

Russian researchers studied the effects of deer horn extract and found that it improved the performance of athletes, but these optimistic results have not been confirmed by clinical studies. Despite the enthusiastic claims of the producers of this remedy, the medical profession is sceptical as to its value. This remedy is, however, popular among Chinese migrants in the West including Australia. Special deer farms have now been established in Australia because of the high demand for this 'rejuvenating' remedy.

Preliminary chemical studies were unable to detect any physiologically active ingredient in this product. We can only state that it does not show any adverse effects.

Deprenyl

The synthetic drug deprenyl is now regarded by some researchers as one of the most potent anti-ageing drugs available. Preliminary tests in experimental animals confirm its life-prolonging potential. Dr. J. Knoll from Semmelweis University of Medicine in Hungary performed his trials using rats. He reported a twofold increase in remaining life expectancy when deprenyl was given to animals at the age of two years. The mechanism of its action is not clear but it is believed that it significantly reduces damage caused by free radicals.

Deprenyl is used in combination with L-dopa to alleviate symptoms of the diseases of old age such as Parkinson's and Alzheimer's disease, and mild improvement has been observed in most patients.

According to some studies deprenyl might also show some anticancer effect by slowing both tumour formation and proliferation. However, more research is needed to confirm these preliminary results.

DHEA

A synthetic version of a human hormone of the adrenal glands called DHEA (dehydroepiandrosterone), is believed by some scientists to be a new wonder drug in the quest for longevity. Its function is still unclear but the level of this hormone in the bloodstream reaches its zenith at the age of about 30 and then gradually declines throughout the rest of life. No other steroidal hormone behaves this way. Some scientists are enthusiastic about the possible benefit of DHEA. According to Dr. Ian Brighthope President of the Australasian College of Nutritional and Environmental Medicine, by taking DHEA a 70-year-old person could in theory prolong their life to 95 years. This view is supported by experiments on animals. It has been found that DHEA inhibits various cancers induced by chemicals. Some studies indicate that the level of this hormone may be linked with breast cancer as women with this disease tend to have low levels of DHEA in their blood. It has also been found that people with below-average levels of DHEA have a higher risk of coronary heart disease.

Research has shown that DHEA plays an important role in brain function, especially by stimulating communication between neurones. Old mice whose memory has been erased by pharmacological means, had their memory restored when given DHEA and their capacity to learn became the same as that of young animals. Clinical studies on the elderly have shown antidepressant action of DHEA and improvement of memory.

DHEA also seems to boost the immune system. When a group of mice were injected with particularly virulent viruses, about 95 percent of these animals died, while those which received DHEA all survived the first virus and 63 percent survived the second. Proponents of the use of the DHEA also claim that it reduces the risk of developing diabetes and such diseases as arthritis and even Alzheimer's disease.

Mainstream doctors still wait for additional clinical studies and consider the therapeutic use of DHEA as premature.

Because of potential adverse effects of DHEA its use is still not permitted in Australia.

DMAE

DMAE (dimethylaminoethanol) is a new synthetic drug which was found to significantly lengthen the life of experimental animals. Richard Hochshind, Scientific Director of the Glenn Foundation for Medical Research in the US, studied the activity of this drug. For a period of time a group of old mice was treated with water in which DMAE was dissolved. To Dr. Hochshind's surprise, the mice that received DMAE lived 50 percent longer than a matched group of mice that did not receive the drug. The drug was also found to improve the learning capacity of old rats. The effects were believed to be caused by inhibiting the formation of the age pigment in their brain cells.

Although no such experiments have so far been performed in humans, many gerontologists already perceive the potential value of DMAE as a life-prolonging agent. The drug is sold in the US. It is used mainly for treating some behavioural problems, especially shortened attention span in children. The drug reaches the brain where it is converted to the neurotransmitter called 'acetylcholine'.

The drug has been tested on patients of various ages and was found to mildly stimulate the central nervous system. Improvements in vitality, alertness and memory were reported in older individuals as a result of long-term treatment. It has been known that in older people the cell-cleansing activity carried out by the tiny bodies called 'lysosomes' is less efficient when the tissue becomes older. Lysosomes are said to become 'crazy' and their capacity to remove waste in brain cells significantly diminishes with age. Consequently, the cells have a tendency to become clogged with harmful deposits. DMAE is believed to improve the capacity of lysosomes to perform their 'cleaning' job and this action may retard the ageing process.

Fo-ti-Tieng

When Chinese Professor Li Chung Yun died in 1933 it was officially announced that he was 256 years old. It was claimed that he outlived his 23 wives and that at the time of his death he was living with his 24th wife. Although such a lifespan cannot be true, he must have lived an exceptionally long life. The secret of this man's longevity is attributed to a herb, Indian marsh pennywort (*Centella asiatica minor*) known in China as Fo-ti-Tieng. It has such a high reputation in China as a rejuvenating medicine that it is called the 'Elixir of Life'.

This plant has a similar reputation in India. It is said that a famous Hindu sage named Nanddo Narian, regularly used this herb to prevent senility and he was feeling young when he reached the age of 107 years. There was a widespread belief in India and Pakistan that all their centenarians regularly used this rejuvenating herbal remedy. In Sri Lanka too, this plant is called a 'longevity plant'. No wonder that Western scientists became interested in this plant.

Among the first to study its properties was the French biochemist Jules Lupin. He found that the plant extract had a stimulating effect on the brain of experimental animals. Professor Mennier of the French Academy of Sciences also studied this plant. He even claimed to have isolated from it a substance showing rejuvenating effects. He called this substance 'The Youth Vitamin X'. He reported that this substance stimulates activity of endocrine glands in animals. He claimed that this plant can be of particular benefit to elderly people as a rejuvenating remedy. His results have so far not been confirmed by other researchers. In fact there are no clinical studies which could show rejuvenating properties of this plant. Despite this, enthusiastic proponents of Fo-ti-Tieng believe that this plant is the "finest of all herbal tonics to treat general debility and decline."

Garlic

Researchers at Loma Linda University School of Medicine in California, studied the physiological properties of garlic compounds. They found that diallyl sulfide found in fresh garlic enhances the efficiency of the immune system in fighting malignancy. In another study, conducted at the Pennsylvania State University, an anticancer effect of garlic was demonstrated. In a group of rats with chemically induced cancer a 70 percent decrease in the size of tumours was observed when the animals were given fresh garlic. A substance recently isolated from garlic by German researchers, called ajoene, inhibits tumour growth in experimental animals. No such studies in humans have so far been performed, but observations of the relationship between garlic intake and incidence of cancer seem to have confirmed its beneficial effects. A study conducted in China involving 1600 individuals revealed that those consuming garlic regularly were up to 60 percent less likely to suffer from stomach cancer when compared with those who did not eat garlic at all.

Research has also confirmed the traditional belief that garlic may prevent coronary heart disease. Epidemiological observations show that in some Mediterranean countries in which fresh garlic is consumed on a daily basis, the rate of heart attacks is significantly lower than in those regions where garlic is less popular. Recent studies have shown that consuming fresh garlic causes gradual lowering of blood cholesterol levels. One gram of garlic extract given daily for six months significantly reduced blood cholesterol in a group of people with elevated blood cholesterol.

Only fresh garlic preparations or fresh garlic must be used since 'deodorised' garlic preparations lose their cholesterol-lowering properties.

Those who want to use fresh garlic instead of an extract to reduce their cholesterol level should realise that up to seven fresh cloves daily must be eaten to achieve the beneficial results. Such large doses of garlic may cause stomach irritation; also, some individuals are allergic to fresh garlic.

Garlic was also found to prevent formation of blood clots and in this way a diet rich in garlic may help prevent heart attack and stroke.

Gerovital

In 1956, Dr. Ana Aslan, a Romanian physician, announced that she had discovered a new rejuvenating remedy she called gerovital. Although it was in fact a well-known anaesthetic called procaine, Dr. Aslan claimed that she could use it successfully as an anti-ageing medicine to rejuvenate elderly patients. It was reported that old and very weak patients left her clinic after a prolonged treatment with gerovital as if they had become 10 years younger. Their arthritic pains disappeared, hearing and vision improved considerably, and in some patients even atherosclerosis had been reversed.

The publicity for her new therapy for the elderly was so effective that her clinic in Bucharest became a world famous rejuvenating centre. Among the first celebrities to become her patients was the 80-year-old Dr. Hewlett Johnson, Dean of Canterbury. He declared: "I had a course of her treatment which has had an extraordinary happy effect on me—restoring powers that I had lost. It made me feel and act as if several years had been taken off my age." Many celebrities from the East and West were among Dr. Aslan's patients. They included Mao Tse-tung, Nikita Khrushchev, Konrad Adenauer, Charles Chaplin and Charles De Gaulle. Initially Dr. Aslan provided testimonials from her enthusiastic patients but there were no clinical double-blind studies performed to evaluate the benefit of the treatment.

In 1972, Dr. Aslan published the results of her study conducted on animals. She found that when old rats were treated with gerovital their life expectancy had increased by over 20 percent when compared with a control groups of animals. These results did not impress scientists in the West because only a small number of animals was used in her experiments. Other scientists could not confirm Dr. Aslan's results. Clinical studies performed in some other European clinics could not show that gerovital was a rejuvenating medicine, although some improvement in the general well-being of elderly patients was noted. Some clinical studies have shown an improvement in learning capacity and in patient mood, especially in depressed individuals. On the other hand, studies in the US and England could only observe some improvement of the skin appearance due to mild dilation of the skin arteries.

Most gerontologists are sceptical and express the view that the 'miraculous' rejuvenating effects of gerovital are solely of a psychological nature.

Dr. Zhores Medvedev, a Russian gerontologist who now lives in England, points out that: "Dr. Aslan transferred very old people from a dull atmosphere of retirement houses to the pleasant atmosphere of her modern clinic and gave them special attention plus 'a miracle drug'; no wonder they felt rejuvenated." Similarly, eminent US gerontologist Dr. Roy L. Walford, is sceptical. He indicates, "No one from this large cohort treated for a long time has broken the maximum lifespan barrier or even come close."

Despite the lack of enthusiasm among Western physicians the use of procaine as a general tonic for elderly patients has survived in some countries In Australia it was prescribed as K.H.3 until 1992.

Ginger

Ginger (*Zingiber officinale*), a popular spice, may be taken as a preventative medicine in the near future. The National Cancer Institute in the United States has recently included ginger in its Experimental Food Program aimed at finding a cancer cure in foods and spices. This interest in the anticancer effect of ginger was initiated by the studies performed at the University of Wisconsin. Charles Ellson investigated the effects of one of the compounds isolated from ginger oil called geraniol. A group of rats with induced cancers was treated with a solution of geraniol and a substantial survival rate was observed in animals who received the treatment.

In another study, geraniol was shown to enhance the tumour-suppressing effects of some prescribed anticancer drugs in experimental animals. No such studies have so far been performed in humans. Ginger has also some blood thinning effect. A diet containing this popular spice was found to inhibit blood cells from sticking together and forming clots, even after a fatty meal. In this way ginger helps prevent heart attack and stroke.

Gingko

Gingko (*Gingko biloba*) is an ancient tree native to Japan and China which has been used for many centuries as a cure for various ailments. Recent studies have shown that an extract from its leaves may be a most useful medicine. It has the power to significantly reduce oedema after stroke, and treatment with gingko extract may gradually lead to a complete restoration of impaired brain function. This effect is of great importance because cerebral oedema is one of the most common diseases in elderly people and a cause of premature death.

Gingko preparations have also been used successfully to prevent thrombosis, dangerous blood clots which may lead to stroke or heart attack. Gingko extracts were also found to improve the blood flow to areas which may be deprived of sufficient blood supply, such as the brain and lower limbs.

Double-blind clinical studies have shown that gingko extracts can help improve memory in some elderly patients. Researchers believe that gingko may therefore be helpful in slowing down some symptoms of ageing. Gingko extracts were shown to be strong free radical scavengers, so they might be helpful with damage involved in the ageing process. A special group of active substances called flavonoids, is responsible for the beneficial effects of gingko preparations.

Various gingko preparations are now available in most Western countries including Australia where they can be obtained in pharmacies and health food stores without prescription. Because of strong pharmacological effects and possible side effects gingko extract should not be used without consulting your doctor.

Ginseng

Ginseng is the most famous Chinese herbal remedy and has been used for over 5000 years. It is the root of a small herbaceous plant (*Panax ginseng*). The root is strange-looking because it often resembles a human body in shape.

Many people in China and Japan believe that ginseng can not only cure many diseases but can also miraculously extend human life.

The Chinese believe that their emperors retained their youthful powers by regular use of the best quality ginseng. Among enthusiastic users of ginseng were Mao, Nehru and Chiang Kai-shek. It has also been used as a rejuvenating medicine by wealthy sheiks of the Middle East and many celebrities in the West.

The properties of the famous medicine were first investigated in Russia, especially by Professor I. I. Brekhman from the Scientific Institute in Vladivostok. He performed many experiments on laboratory animals and obtained beneficial results. A group of mice was fed ginseng and their capacity to swim was compared with a control group of animals. Mice that received ginseng were found to swim for almost twice as long as the mice in the control group. Thus, it has been shown that ginseng increased stamina and considerably improved physical performance. Russian scientists have also revealed that ginseng extract given to rats prolonged their lifespan.

Many studies conducted in the West have shown beneficial effects of ginseng in treating elderly patients. In order to eliminate the placebo effect, neither doctors nor patients knew which preparation contained ginseng. Among those elderly patients who received ginseng, general improvement in mood and activity was observed. In addition, increased personal initiative and improved memory and concentration were also noted. Researchers concluded that ginseng "was suitable for counteracting the general falling off of physical and mental abilities that is the first symptom of old age."

Perhaps the most extensive clinical study on the effect of ginseng treatment was performed by Dr. U. J. Schmidt in Germany. Ginseng extracts were given to 540 elderly patients for a long period of time and their condition was observed. In almost all patients treated, their mood, drive and ability to concentrate significantly improved when compared to a group that received placebo.

There is no proof yet that ginseng can cure any specific disease, but it may speed recovery by stimulating the body's own capacity to heal itself. The claim that ginseng can prolong human lifespan is hard to test because such a study would take so long. However, despite the fact that there is insufficient evidence that ginseng can extend human life, studies involving elderly people indicate that ginseng can produce increased vitality during ageing. Some studies show that ginseng is also a stress-relieving remedy and that it may help an older person to resist some of the effects of increasing age, by making the body better able to ward off infection.

Scientists of the Kanazawa University in Japan have recently found that certain ginseng substances called saponins have anti-tumour effects. These substances inhibited the growth of cancer cells in a culture. They were even capable of transforming malignant cells back into normal cells. These results have not yet been confirmed by other researchers.

According to Dr. C. Liu from China, ginseng contains 28 different ginsenosides, which were found to act favourably on the cardiovascular system and to stimulate endocrine secretion. In addition, these substances were found to improve the function of the immune system, relieve stress and "have an anti-ageing effect." In a report published in the 1992 *Journal of Ethnopharmacology*, Dr. Liu indicates that substances isolated from ginseng "prevent the shrinkage of the adrenal gland due to ageing."

Ginseng also lowers blood cholesterol levels and improves the cholesterol–HDL ratio. Ginseng is generally a safe remedy, but in some individuals it may increase blood pressure and cause insomnia. People who have asthma or suffer from emphysema should avoid taking this remedy because their condition may deteriorate.

Ginseng is hard to grow and it is among the most expensive natural products. It is often adulterated with roots of other plants. In fact, tests conducted in England have shown that some ginseng preparations had only traces of the genuine ginseng.

Another plant which has similar effects is *Eleutherococcus senticosus*, called Siberian ginseng. It is used in China and Russia as a tonic. The plant has a similar action to genuine ginseng. When the extract of this plant was given to athletes their performance was much better when compared with a control group. In a test performed with mice, those who received the extract of the plant could swim for 33 percent longer than the untreated mice. Since 1962 preparations of Siberian ginseng have been approved as an official tonic for elderly people in Russia.

Honey bee pollen

The use of honey bee pollen dates back to ancient times. Ancient texts from Egypt and Persia refer to it. Greek philosophers claimed that bee pollen held the secret of eternal youth. It was used, together with honey, by the early Olympic athletes to get extra energy and vitality.

Pollen is said to be a treasure house of nutrition and regenerative powers. It contains 19 amino acids, all the vitamins, plus certain hormones and enzymes. Bee pollen is the richest source of rutin which strengthens capillaries. DNA and RNA are also found in large quantities in pollen.

Bee pollen is the richest natural source of vitamin B_6. This vitamin helps to break down homocysteine, a toxic substance which appears to play a role in developing coronary heart disease. According to the Physician's Health Study, people with the highest levels of homocysteine in their blood are three times more likely to suffer from heart attack than those with lower levels of this substance. Researchers have recently found that depletion of vitamin B_6 in elderly people can cause depression of the immune system. Release of interleukin-2 and the production of lymphocytes which follows, increases the efficiency of immune system.

Russian gerontologists, N. Mankovsky and D.G. Chebotarev, claim that honey bee pollen is a rejuvenating agent capable of extending human life. This claim has so far not been substantiated by any scientific evidence.

In various trials it has been shown that bee pollen increases athletic performance and combats fatigue. In 1976, the Finnish track coach talked about his country's Olympic team and revealed the following: "Most of our athletes take bee pollen supplements. Our studies show that it significantly improves their performance." Similarly, the British Olympic coach asserted: "At least 90% of our athletes take bee pollen. Of all those I've tested, I believe it's the most effective natural food of its kind available to athletes today."

Hormone replacement therapy

Among users of hormone replacement therapy (HRT), some studies have found the rate of heart attack to be reduced when compared with the general population. Many women opt for hormone replacement therapy to alleviate unpleasant menopausal symptoms. There is some concern about the safety of such therapy because the use of oestrogen has been linked with an increased risk of ovarian cancer. A study of 240,000 women sponsored by the American Cancer Society has revealed that there is such a risk. Women who took oestrogen regularly for six years had a 40 percent increased risk of developing lethal ovarian cancer. In women who took such treatment for 11 years or more, the risk increased up to 70 percent. Researchers, however, point out that today's risk must be much lower because the normal dose used before was 1.25 mg of oestrogen and currently it is only 0.625 mg. The risk of contracting ovarian cancer has been further reduced by modifying the therapy, combining oestrogen with progestine.

Many women also worry that HRT causes an increased risk of breast cancer. According to Professor A. MacLennan of the University of Adelaide, there is no convincing research evidence anywhere in the world to attest that hormone replacement therapy can be considered a risk factor linked to breast cancer. There was only one highly publicised study which suggested an increase in breast cancer among women who use hormone replacement therapy for five years or longer. Another study, however, showed no increase in breast cancer and actually suggested there was a reduction in breast cancer in women who used this therapy for eight years or more. We will have to wait until 2005, when the results of a large, long-term study become known, before we will be sure about the safety of HRT.

Huangqi

Two medicinal plants (*Astragalus membraceous* and *Ligustrum lucidum*) are used in China as a remedy called huangqi. Chinese doctors claim that these plants stimulate a weakened immune system, cure various diseases and have particular value as a rejuvenating remedy for elderly people. Huangqi is one of the most popular herbal medicines in China.

According to a report of the Chinese Academy of Medical Sciences, these plants are used by Chinese practitioners of traditional medicine in about 40 percent of all prescriptions. Currently in China these herbs are given to cancer patients. In a special treatment, known as Fu-zheng Therapy, which is practised in many Chinese hospitals, these herbs are used to treat cancer along with chemotherapy and radiotherapy. In a clinical trial which involved some 1000 cancer patients, survival times of the patients who received Fu-zheng treatment with herbs nearly doubled when compared with the control group of patients. According to Chinese scientists, extracts of these plants boost the ability of the immune system to fight cancer. The promising curative effects of Huangqi have so far not been confirmed by Western researchers.

Kerosene

Kerosene has traditionally been used in Russia and in some East European countries as a remedy to treat cancer. It has also been recommended as a preventive measure against cancer and as a life-prolonging cure. This remedy is also used occasionally in Australia. Some cancer patients refuse the treatment prescribed by their doctors and instead put their trust in kerosene therapy. As this substance has no anticancer action, such 'unusual treatment' cannot be effective. When the disappointed patient finally returns to modern treatment, it is often too late as the disease has progressed because of unnecessary delay in treatment.

The internal use of kerosene is not only useless, it is also hazardous. Prolonged use of kerosene may lead to serious poisoning. Irreversible liver or kidney damage may occur. The use of kerosene in larger doses may be fatal.

In Australia some people also use kerosene-containing lotions as a treatment for rheumatic pain. They are advised to use such a lotion by irresponsible naturopaths who are ready to supply 'the wonderful remedy' to their patients by postal order. In one case, an Adelaide woman used such a lotion for a few weeks. She received no pain relief but soon started suffering itching to her skin. She noticed that the area of skin was covered with small furuncles. She consulted a medical doctor who ordered her to stop using the lotion. The symptoms disappeared. It is well known that kerosene used topically has a strong irritating action on the skin and mucous membranes, and prolonged use may cause severe skin damage.

In fact not only kerosene but also mineral oils are hazardous, especially when used internally. Benign pulmonary lesions were observed in some elderly people who habitually used mineral oils such as paraffin as a laxative.

Kombucha tea

Kombucha tea is brewed from a culture of what is called a 'Kombucha fungus'. Actually it is not a fungus but a symbiotic association of yeasts (*Saccharomycodes ludwigii*) and certain bacteria. The 'fungus' is usually grown on a mixture of ordinary cold tea and sugar. It is believed to be a cure for a whole range of ailments including cancer as well as a general tonic and remedy for promoting longevity. Kombucha tea is highly popular among centenarians in China, Russia and the Ukraine. There is, however, no evidence that people who regularly use it live longer.

In Australia this 'fungus' is available in local health food stores. People who use Kombucha tea noted a general feeling of well-being, lack of tiredness and the sensation of being more alert. In Germany, some cancer specialists tried this remedy on cancer patients and there were claims that in some cases the therapy was highly successful. However, there are at present no clinical studies which could support this contention. The proponents of this therapy claim that patients suffering from arthritis who have undergone Kombucha tea therapy had less swelling in the joints, less pain and increased mobility. Unfortunately, when they stopped taking the tea, the pain returned.

A number of AIDS patients took Kombucha tea and they had more energy, but medical doctors did not notice any measurable improvement in their immune system nor a difference in the T-cell counts.

Kombucha tea contains glucuronic and L-lactic acids, vitamin B and traces of heparin, the drug which is used to prevent blood clots. Some people are sensitive to Kombucha tea and the side effects include: constipation, mild diarrhoea, rashes and even sores on the mouth, nausea, dizziness and fatigue. Some children have experienced sleeplessness. Pregnant or lactating women should not use it.

Laetril

One of the remedies that is supposed to cure cancer is laetril, also known as vitamin B_{17}. Laetril is not a vitamin. It is obtained from the seeds of the apricot (*Prunus armenica*). The main ingredient of this medicine is a substance called amygdalin which, in the human body, causes the release of hydrocyanic acid that is claimed to be the anticancer agent.

Proponents of laetril therapy maintain that it selectively destroys tumour cells leaving the healthy cells intact. However, in experiments on laboratory animals which were given laetril and had chemically induced cancers, no decrease in malignant growth could be observed. Furthermore, reports from the US physicians who collected data about some 1000 cancer patients who used laetril have revealed that the treatment had no curative effects. As there was still great public demand for more investigation of laetril, a special study was performed at the National Cancer Institute in the US. In this clinical study 178 cancer patients were treated with laetril for a specific period of time and their conditions observed. There was no difference in mortality rate between the group of patients who received laetril and those who received placebo. The proponents of laetril therapy based their claims for the medicine's benefits on patient testimonials which cannot be clinically confirmed. In the meantime, severe cases of poisoning in patients who used laetril began to appear, especially in the US. Some people died as a result of prolonged laetril use. This medicine is now banned in the USA, Australia and most European countries. Despite this evident hazard and lack of proven benefit, some people in Australia demand that this 'medicine' should be available as they believe in its miraculous power to conquer cancer.

Maitake

Maitake mushroom (*Grifola frondosa*) is found in north-eastern Japan. For hundreds of years Japanese herbalists recommended this mushroom for strengthening the body and improving overall health. Recent studies have confirmed some of these assumptions. It has been found that maitake mushroom can improve many functions of the immune system that helps in fighting disease. Preliminary studies conducted in the United States show that this mushroom inhibits induction of colorectal cancer in experimental animals. The results of these studies have so far not been confirmed in humans.

Melatonin

Melatonin is not available in Australia but it is available in New Zealand and the USA. It is a hormone produced by the pineal gland of the brain during sleep. It plays an important role in maintaining normal body rhythms, particularly the sleep–wake cycle. It is also believed to be of vital importance in maintaining various other body functions. It has been observed that secretions of melatonin significantly decrease with age so it was speculated that it may have influence over the ageing process.

An interesting experiment has been performed by Italian scientist, Dr. Walter Pierpaoli and his colleagues. They used two groups of mice, 10 old and 10 young mice. Their pineal glands were swapped, that is, the old mice received young pineal glands while the young mice received old pineal glands. All mice were genetically identical so the transplants could not be rejected. It was found that young mice with old pineal glands began to die much earlier than would normally be expected, while the old mice with young pineal glands lived 20 percent longer than their normal life expectancy.

Other studies with experimental animals that had their pineal glands removed, have also shown an accelerated ageing process.

In a review article in the *International Journal of Neuroscience* (1990) written by Reuben Sandyk of the Albert Einstein College of Medicine, the value of melatonin was discussed: "There is evidence from both experimental animal and human studies to suggest a decreased melatonin function may accelerate the ageing process and thus support the notion that melatonin may function as an anti-ageing hormone."

Scientific evidence about the potential anti-ageing effect in humans is still scarce and there are only testimonials from those elderly people who used this hormone as a rejuvenating medicine. Eighty percent of these patients reported increased vitality while 12 percent did not see any improvement in their health condition.

So far, all researchers agree that melatonin can be an effective agent to treat insomnia. Because of great public interest in the hormone, a special research group has recently been set up in the US to study melatonin's safety and effectiveness as a medicine. Meanwhile three to five million Americans take melatonin regularly in the belief that it will rejuvenate them.

Nucleic acids

There are two essential nucleic acids—DNA (deoxyribonucleic acid) and RNA (ribonucleic acid)—both present in the nucleus of every body cell. These acids are necessary for the formation of new cells, cell repair processes and cell metabolism. When we are young new cells grow very quickly, but as we age the replacement of old cells slows down. Some researchers believe that the ageing process may be partly caused by decline in the level or capacity of these important nucleic acids. It is assumed by some scientists that if the lost nucleic acids are replenished we may be able to restrict the ageing process.

These suggestions have been confirmed by recent studies. According to one recent study reported in the *Journal of the American Geriatric Society*, diet supplemented with nucleic acids increases the life expectancy of experimental animals. One group of mice was given weekly injections of a mixture of DNA and RNA while another group remained untreated. The mice that received these supplements were found to live twice as long as the control group. The treated mice were also more alert and looked healthier. These preliminary results in animals have not yet been confirmed in clinical studies.

Some people have already turned to nucleic acid supplements which can be obtained from health food stores. Although taking such supplements is safe, some precautions should be taken. Nucleic acids taken in excess may considerably increase uric acid levels and produce gout in susceptible individuals. People who have a tendency to develop gout should not only abstain from taking such supplements, but should avoid foods rich in these acids. Nucleic acids occur in large amounts in many foods such as mushrooms, spinach, asparagus and wheat germ.

Pega Palo

In the mid-1950s it was reported in the United States that a certain plant called Pega Palo, growing on the island of Dominica in the Caribbean, is a strong rejuvenating herb. It was claimed that this remedy could turn an 80-year-old man into a 30-year-old one. It was believed that this plant had the power to restore normal function in the sex glands of elderly men.

Visitors to Dominica were offered the preparation made from Pega Palo and sold in the form of a tincture in small bottles for about five dollars. Many tourists who experimented with the tincture noted remarkable 'rejuvenating' effects. Because of increased publicity, soon many businesses were established supplying Americans with the famous remedy. In fact Pega Palo became very popular in the US.

Pega Palo was found not to be a single plant species but there is still some uncertainty as to its actual composition. The distributors of the tincture label it as either containing the plants belonging to *Rhynchosia* or *Paulinia* species. The first plants *R pyramidalis* and *R. serpentina* are suspected to have hallucinogenic effects while *Paulinia sorbilis* and *P. cupana* are known to contain caffeine in their seeds.

The pharmacological properties of the tincture were examined in animals (rats). It had no effect on the size or weight of testes nor did it influence the prostate gland. Researchers could in fact not establish any pronounced physiological properties of the tincture so it seems that the claimed rejuvenating or aphrodisiac effects of Pega Palo are without scientific foundation.

Placenta tissue therapy

Placenta tissue therapy is the brainchild of Professor V. P. Filatov, a Soviet ophthalmologist who became famous for his corneal transplantation developed in the 1930s. Professor Filatov noticed that when the cornea graft was stored in a cold environment for some time before transplantation, such grafts were much better accepted than grafts using fresh corneas. He speculated that by freezing tissues, special substances are formed which he called biostimulants. After experimenting with various tissues he eventually decided to choose the placenta. He claimed that because placenta covers the embryo it must contain a variety of stimulants that could be used as a cure for various ailments.

He treated elderly patients with his new cure and claimed general improvement in their health. He noticed improved physical performance, improved skin appearance and increased sexual power of most of the treated patients for a period of up to 10 years. He also claimed that he could observe a typical reversal of ageing symptoms in many elderly patients.

The beneficial effects of this therapy were not confirmed by the Western scientists who performed double-blind studies on elderly patients. Neither could they confirm the existence of biostimulating substances in frozen placenta tissue.

Despite this evident lack of scientific basis, the use of placenta therapy has survived in some countries. In France, for example, a sterile placenta extract has been used for intramuscular injections, and producers of this preparation—known as Placentaphil—not only claim it to have strong healing effects, but also claim that it acts by retarding symptoms of ageing. Most gerontologists remain sceptical. As Dr. Saul Kent points out: "It is possible that the observed improvements in function were largely or entirely due to the effects of diet, exercise or some other factors. It could be that the attention given to the patients contributed substantially."

Reishi

Some 2500 years ago a Chinese emperor ordered his men to travel around the world in search of a 'mushroom of immortality'. The mushroom they found was *Ganoderma lucidum*, called ling chih in China and reishi in Japan.

In Japan, reishi is officially recognised as enhancing cancer treatment, and it also has a reputation as a longevity herb. It has been used as a general tonic and to fight infection. In Japan people use reishi to treat liver disease, atherosclerosis and hypertension. It is a popular remedy in China, where it is used in about 30 percent of all herbal preparations.

The anti-tumour effects of reishi are claimed to be based on the presence of certain polysaccharides that enhance the ability of the immune system to fight disease. Reishi was also found to have antioxidant effects thus lowering the risk of many diseases.

Royal jelly

Many people believe that royal jelly contains the secret of longevity. This is because royal jelly is the only food of the queen bee which has an incredible lifespan when compared with worker bees. The queen bee is the only member of the hive that is fed royal jelly during her entire life. She lives for up to six years, that is, 72 times longer than worker bees.

Royal jelly was found to contain a number of physiologically active ingredients such as hormone-like substances, enzymes and various vitamins. It is particularly rich in pantothenic acid, one of the vitamin Bs. In fact, it contains six times more pantothenic acid than liver and brewer's yeast.

Royal jelly was found to increase the lifespan of fruit flies. Researchers assume that this effect is caused by the presence of the pantothenic acid in royal jelly. When pure pantothenic acid was given to mice, about a 20 percent increase in life expectancy was observed. Together with choline, pantothenic acid is involved in the formation of the major neurotransmitter, acetylcholine, and decline of this neurotransmitter is known to lead to senility symptoms in elderly people. Small wonder that some gerontologists consider pantothenic acid to be an agent which might delay symptoms of ageing. Some physicians already advise their elderly patients to use pantothenic acid supplements on a daily basis.

A five-year-long Czechoslovakian study of the effects of royal jelly on elderly people showed its beneficial effects on atherosclerosis. In most patients with high cholesterol, blood cholesterol levels were also lowered.

In recent years some naturopaths have recommended royal jelly as a natural remedy to cure cancer. This claim is probably based on a scientific report published in *Cancer Research* in 1960. It describes an experiment in which a group of mice was inoculated with cancer cells. Half the group received royal jelly as a food, the other half was kept on ordinary food. All mice fed with royal jelly survived while those in the control group all died of cancer. It was concluded that royal jelly had a pronounced anticancer effect in animals. Unfortunately, no clinical studies were conducted to confirm these promising results.

Although royal jelly can be regarded as generally safe, some people may be strongly allergic to this product. In 1993, a young girl who was given royal jelly as a tonic suffered a serious asthma attack and died. Fortunately such cases are rare. To avoid a potential fatality each product containing royal jelly has a warning on its label.

Shiitake

The Chinese consider the shiitake mushroom (*Lentinus edodes*) to be one of the most beneficial natural remedies. For many centuries, eating this mushroom was recommended for strengthening a weak immune system as well as for preventing various ailments. Chinese legends glorify this mushroom as a plant that has the power to bring eternal youth.

Recent Japanese studies have shown that some of these claims have a scientific basis. A compound called lentinan was isolated from shiitake and found to have some beneficial effects. It stimulates the production of T-lymphocytes and interleukins. This discovery is of vital importance since it is well known that interleukins can destroy malignant cells and kill viruses.

Further investigation has confirmed the anti-tumour action of the shiitake extract. It was found to suppress the action of cancer-inducing substances in experimental animals and to inhibit the spread of tumours. It was then observed that such action is most beneficial after surgical removal of tumours. Shiitake mushroom, when given to patients, was found to extend their lifespan after surgery in advanced stomach, colorectal and breast cancer.

Some researchers believes that shiitake mushrooms may be helpful in fighting AIDS. Dr. S. Sarker claims that a shiitake mushroom extract may block the replication of the AIDS virus, especially in the late stages of the disease (*Antiviral Research*, 1993).

Urinotherapy

It may seem incredible but in some regions of the world the drinking of one's own urine is regarded as a remedy for maintaining good health. There is a common belief in India and Taiwan that drinking urine can not only prevent or cure many diseases but can also prolong life. In the ancient Yogic scripts *Damara Tantra*, a special technique is described which is called 'urine revitalising technique'. Nor is urine drinking popular only in rural areas among uneducated people. Prominent politicians were among those who regularly drank their urine to keep well. Mahatma Gandhi, former Prime Minister of India, was said to have drunk his urine daily in a belief that it would prolong his life. Drinking urine as a cure for any ailment is popular in Taiwan. It is said that to keep well and prolong life, up to 200,000 Taiwanese drink their urine every day. Taiwan even has a special 'Urine Therapy Hot Line'.

In some rural regions of Russia drinking urine is considered to be a useful self-treatment for many diseases including rheumatism and cancer. Even today some healers recommend this treatment to their patients. This technique even has its official name, 'uropathy'. Patients are often advised not only to drink their own urine regularly, but also to squirt it into various body orifices.

Urine has been considered to be completely devoid of any physiologically active ingredients. Recently however, traces of the hormone melatonin have been found to be present in urine. The concentration of this hormone in urine is so low that it is unlikely that it can have any pronounced effect.

Yoghurt

Dr. Ilya Metchnikoff (1845–1916), a famous Russian bacteriologist and Nobel Prize winner for Medicine, believed that ageing is mainly caused by bacteria. He claimed that toxins produced by bacteria living in the intestine gradually poison the whole body, causing accelerated ageing. To prevent this he recommended change in the intestinal bacterial flora by consuming a lot of yoghurt. This, he claimed, would make the large intestine "too acidic" for harmful bacteria to survive.

To support his theory, Metchnikoff pointed out that Bulgaria had so many centenarians because they all had a yoghurt-rich diet. Further studies, however, did not confirm Metchnikoff's theory. We know now that bacteria found in the large intestine are not harmful, and people who had their large intestine surgically removed did not live longer.

Recent studies however, show that a diet rich in yoghurt may be beneficial to our health. According to a study conducted at the University of California in 1992, people who ate a diet rich in yoghurt had a four times higher concentration of interferons than the groups who received placebo. Since interferons are antiviral agents, this study indicates that yoghurt may enhance our resistance to infections.

Chapter Seven

RECENT DEVELOPMENTS AND FUTURE BREAKTHROUGHS

Gene therapy

History shows that there have been three great revolutions in the development of our ability to prevent or treat diseases. The first was the establishment of sanitation systems which protected a vast number of people from fatal infections. The second revolution occurred with the introduction of surgery under anaesthesia; for the first time this enabled doctors to save people affected by illnesses previously regarded as incurable. The third great leap forward took place with the development of vaccines and antibiotics which helped to prevent many lethal diseases caused by bacteria.

Gene therapy will be the fourth revolution in medicine because delivery of selected genes into a patient's cells has the potential to cure the vast majority of diseases, including many that have so far resisted treatment. The rapid development of genetic science confirmed the suspicion that almost every illness is caused in part because one or more genes are not functioning properly. Such defective genes order our cells to produce improper proteins, causing disease. More than 4000 human diseases are known to be caused by inborn damage to a single gene. Many illnesses such as coronary heart disease, arthritis and senility are caused to some extent by impairment of one or more genes involved in body defence systems. Liver cells, for example, manufacture proteins that help clear cholesterol from our blood. An imperfect gene responsible for this function leads to a reduction in the amount or efficiency of this protein, leading to high blood cholesterol levels, atherosclerosis and coronary heart disease.

Although at present our understanding of the precise genetic origin of many diseases is sketchy, this knowledge is expected to increase enormously in the next few decades. By the year 2000, it is assumed that scientists working on the Human Genome Project will be able to determine the chromosomal location of nearly all active human genes. Researchers will also study the function of each detected gene, making it possible to identify all those gene malfunctions which cause disease.

At present, in a number of medical centres around the world trials are being performed aimed at a new treatment called gene therapy. The first patient treated in this revolutionary way was a four-year-old girl from the United States, Ashanti DeSilva. Her treatment commenced on 14 September, 1990. She was suffering from an incurable deficiency of the immune system which resulted from a defective gene she inherited from each of her parents. The normal gene is responsible for the production of an enzyme required for proper functioning of the immune system. With the defective gene, Ashanti was extremely vulnerable to any infection and had to be kept in isolation.

In this treatment white blood cells were removed from her body, normal copies of the defective gene were inserted into them, and then the modified cells were returned to her bloodstream. The results of this treatment were dramatic. She soon recovered and with the help of occasional booster treatment she became a healthy young child.

Researchers have developed several methods of transporting genetic material. In the most effective technique modified viruses are used as gene carriers. The viruses were chosen because they are able to penetrate cells and insert the genetic material into the cells of the new host. But before viruses can be used in gene therapy, their own genes, which are responsible for their reproduction and cause disease in humans, must be removed and replaced with the corrective gene. In this way the virus can be used for transporting proper genes into human cells. The modified virus is in fact identical to the original virus on the outside but is now harmless.

Clinical trials of gene therapy relating to the treatment of many diseases have been conducted with promising results. It has recently been reported in the United States for instance, that gene therapy has shrunk tumours in lung-cancer patients. In an experiment conducted at the M. D. Anderson Cancer Center in Houston, scientists injected healthy copies of a tumour-suppressing gene called p53 into cells that had lost them. Defects in the p53 gene are said to be responsible for 60 percent of cancer cases.

Longevity genes

It has long been speculated that longevity genes do exist, but no evidence to support this had been provided by researchers. In 1993 a significant discovery was made. Dr. Thomas E. Johnson from the University of Colorado isolated a single mutation of a gene he called the age-1 or apo-E gene. He was able to find this gene in nematodes, a species of unsegmented worm which live in garden soil. He established that those worms that have the normal version of the age-1 gene have a maximum lifespan, that is, they live for 37 days. On the other hand, those worms that carry two copies of the mutant age-1 gene have a maximum lifespan twice as long as the ordinary worms of this species.

Nematodes are, however, very simple animals with only about 1 percent of the total number of genes found in humans. It appears logical to assume that in humans there must be a much larger number of genes which are responsible for our longevity. Every human cell has about 100,000 genes.

We know now that in humans there are three variants of the apogene, namely E2, E3 and E4. Everybody inherits one E gene from each parent. More than half the human population carry two E3 genes. People who have the longest life expectancy are those who have two E2 genes, while those with two E4 genes have the shortest lifespan. It has been found that people who carry the E2 genes are about four times more likely to live longer and attain the age of 100 years than those who were born with an E4 gene. Researchers now maintain that the presence of the E4 gene signifies a risk of Alzheimer's disease and heart disease. Studies have revealed that middle-aged women with an E4 gene have twice the risk of coronary heart disease that the rest of the population has, while men who carry the E4 gene have a 50 percent higher risk. Among Americans with Alzheimer's disease, two-thirds have at least one E4 gene; by contrast, only 15 percent of the rest of the population have one E4 gene.

Researchers believe that it is now possible to determine an individual's lifespan from a simple blood test. When the exact role of the E2 gene in controlling our lifespan is established, a treatment may eventually be discovered based on its properties.

Genes, however, appear not to be the only factor which determines an individual's lifespan. Danish researchers examined the lifespan of every pair of identical twins born in that country between 1870 and 1910. Identical twins have the same genes. The study showed an average difference of 14.5 years in their lifespan. This study indicates that factors other than genetics must also have a strong influence in determining an individual's lifespan.

Gene against obesity

Researchers at the Rockefeller University in New York isolated a gene preventing over-eating in mice of normal weight. It is called Ob gene (from the word 'obesity'). The gene is responsible for the production of a protein known as leptin. This protein was obtained in large quantity by inserting the Ob gene into a bacterium. Because bacteria reproduce quickly, the gene was also copied and soon the scientists had a sufficient amount of leptin produced on the basis of information contained in the gene.

Protein obtained in such an unusual way was then injected into the obese mice for a period of one month. As a result, the mice lost 40 percent of their weight.

In the case of humans, probably more than one gene is linked to obesity; nevertheless, we can hope that in the future these genes will be identified and the obesity problems of many people will be solved, thereby extending their lifespan. In such a way the lifespan of many people could be extended.

Artificial genes

Rapid development of genetic science in the last decade has enabled scientists to isolate many genes and determine their structure. For example, a specific gene has been isolated from certain bacteria called *Esherichia coli*. Once this gene was isolated using an electron microscope, it was possible to take a picture of the gene. This further enabled researchers to study this gene in detail. They were able to determine the precise number of nucleotides, the structural units of nucleic acids that form this particular gene. Having obtained all this detailed information, the researchers at the Massachusetts Institute of Technology succeeded in producing the first artificial gene. They made it by linking up its 126 nucleotides in the correct sequence. This artificial gene was fully functional. When inserted into this kind of bacterium it treated this gene as if it were a natural part of its cell.

In early 1996, researchers at the Johns Hopkins University, Baltimore, developed an artificial gene which can be used to fight cancer. When such a gene is introduced into the culture of malignant tissue, the gene seeks out the malignant cells and destroys them. When the gene contacts the protein of the cancer cell it produces a toxic enzyme which kills the cancer cell. When this artificial gene is introduced to a culture with normal cells, the toxic enzyme is not produced; this is because it is only triggered by proteins in the cancer cells.

Phoney viruses and vaccines

Nir Kossovsky and co-workers at the University of California created the so-called phoney viruses which can be used as a vaccine to prevent some diseases. Preliminary results indicate that the phoney virus can even cause some immune responses against AIDS.

A phoney virus is created by taking surface proteins of a virus, removing the infectious core, and replacing that genetic core with a ceramic core. The proteins then reassemble themselves on the ceramic. When the phoney virus is injected, the body's immune system 'believes' it to be an infectious agent. Consequently, when the real and hazardous virus invades the body, its immune system is already prepared to fight and win the battle and thus prevent the disease.

The same principle is used with present day vaccines; instead of a phoney virus however, detoxified viruses are injected. This method has its drawbacks. In some cases the body does not recognise the deactivated virus, or the deactivated virus may still prove to be harmful.

Cryonics

Members of the so-called Cryonics Society in the US believe that at death, or shortly before legal death, an individual should be frozen in liquid nitrogen and then stored until a cure for the disease that caused death can be found. When a cure is available, they argue, the individual's body would be thawed, revived and treated. He or she would then resume normal living.

Until recently, most scientists regarded this reasoning as pure science fiction with no chance of becoming reality. It was thought that even individual organs could not be stored at very low temperatures and later revived. The dream of storing organs at very low temperatures had been hampered by the damage inflicted on cell membranes by water which expands as it freezes.

Now, researchers at the University of Pretoria in South Africa claim to have solved the problem with a new 'cryoprotectant' liquid which is non-toxic, does not rupture cells as it freezes, and exerts little osmotic pressure across cell membranes. These scientists have completed the resuscitation of a rat's heart that had been frozen to –196°C. They soak a rat's heart in cryoprotectant and freeze it in liquid nitrogen. When thawed out, the revived heart beats normally and shows no signs of cellular damage under the electron microscope. The team has also revived frozen rat livers and kidneys. Even rat brains seem to survive freezing unharmed, although they have only undergone structural tests and not tests to check whether they work properly.

However, there still appear to be insurmountable problems when it comes to freezing an entire human body. There are thousands of different types of cells in the human body, and they would probably require different rates of freezing and thawing to remain viable. Thus, it seems that freezing and thawing a whole body at a single rate, as is currently done, would probably not lead to the survival of most cell types. However, a solution to this problem may be found in the future.

Rejuvenating the human brain

Some people speculate that when we reach advanced age we might remain generally healthy but that our mental capacity may be so low that we will be like zombies. This will not necessarily be the case.

Researchers at the University of Rochester's Center for Brain Research discovered that brain cells can be transplanted among animals. Foetal brain cells from one strain of rat were transplanted into the brains of adult rats belonging to another strain. The transplanted cells functioned normally, correcting brain defects. Scientists speculate that in the future it may be possible to rejuvenate ageing human brains. By taking brain-cell transplants, an individual's memory and intelligence could be improved and stroke damage could be reversed.

Scientists at the Centre for Brain Repair in Cambridge are currently investigating the possibility of culturing embryonic brain cells in order to obtain an almost unlimited supply of tissue for transplants. As Clive Svendsen, the research team leader, explains: "Our ultimate goal is to be able to take a single embryo and grow sufficient cells from it to provide transplants for one thousand patients." Brain cell grafts might one day help people with Parkinson's disease or other incurable diseases such as multiple sclerosis.

Artificial organs

Scientists have already successfully constructed artificial tissues that look and function like their natural counterparts. This has been possible because of profound advances in cell biology and plastic manufacture. Scientists can now use ultra pure, biodegradable plastics. With the help of computer design they shape plastics into complicated scaffolding beds that imitate the structure of particular tissues and even organs. The scaffolds are then treated with compounds that will assist cells to adhere and multiply. Finally, these scaffolds are 'seeded' with cells. The seeded cells begin to divide and assemble and the plastic degrades. Eventually only coherent tissue remains. The new permanent tissue can then be implanted in the patient's body.

This technique has already been tried in animals, e.g. when artificial heart valves were engineered in lambs using cells taken from the animal's blood vessels.

For several years, human skin grown on plastics has been grafted onto burnt people and to the foot ulcers of diabetics, with some success.

In the future, whole organs such as livers and kidneys will be obtained in this way; that is, designed, manufactured and transferred to patients. The surgeon will only need to connect it with the patient's blood vessels, nerves and lymph channels.

This method will also be used to repair damage to joints and bones.

In the future, even arms and hands will be made of artificial tissues. The structure of the entire system would be duplicated in biodegradable plastic. It would take about six weeks to grow the arm and then it would be attached to the body. The only current problem is regeneration of nerve tissues. Up to now, no-one has succeeded in growing human nerve cells but many scientists are confident this problem will eventually be overcome. However, before this is accomplished, microelectronic devices may be substituted for implants of engineered nervous tissue.

Antiangiogenic therapy

Drugs that fight cancer by blocking blood supply to tumours are currently undergoing initial clinical trials. The drugs block angiogenesis, that is, the formation of fresh blood vessels. Angiogenesis enables tumours to obtain their own blood supply.

Many inhibitors and potential inhibitors are under study in various university laboratories and biotechnology companies around the world. The most promising compound is a protein called angiostatin which was discovered in mouse urine by Michael O'Reilly at the Children's Hospital Medical Center in Boston. In animals, angiostatin has been shown to stop nearly all blood vessel growth in a large tumour. In laboratory experiments, human breast, colon and prostate cancers have been implanted in mice and allowed to grow to 1 percent of the animal's body weight. When angiostatin was administered, the tumours were reduced to microscopic size and held in a dormant state for as long as the drug was given. Angiostatin only stops the multiplication of endothelial cells, that is, it does not affect other cells. Researchers have not found any toxic effects of angiostatin and the animals do not appear to develop any resistance to the drug.

Investigators at the Cancer Institute in Boston have found that, in laboratory animals, a combination of angiogenesis inhibitors and chemotherapeutic drugs is more effective than chemotherapy alone. In one case, 42 percent of the animals were cured by a combination of treatments but not by either therapy alone.

The above developments could lead not only to finding a cancer treatment but also to treatment of other angiogenic diseases such as blindness caused by the growth of unwanted blood vessels in the eyes of the elderly and people with diabetes.

Organ transplants

Scientists envisage that in the foreseeable future animal organs could be used to replace our malfunctioning, injured or worn out organs. At present it is extremely difficult and often impossible to find a suitable human donor and many people die as a result.

To make the animal organs suitable for transplantation we would breed genetically altered animals by incorporating certain human genes into animals' chromosomes.

Pigs are now on the verge of providing humans with organs suitable for human transplant. In 1992, a British biotechnology company called Imutran succeeded in breeding a pig named "Astrid" which had been genetically engineered to carry certain genes from the human immune system. Researchers believed that this technique would be extremely helpful in overcoming the rejection processes which destroy the recipient's organs within an hour of receiving the transplant.

Initial trials are encouraging. Hearts from genetically altered pigs have been transplanted into monkeys which were treated with immunosuppressive drugs. After transplant, the hearts from genetically engineered pigs were beating in the bodies of two monkey recipients for more than 60 days. In monkeys which received a transplant of an ordinary pig's heart, these organs lasted only an hour before they were destroyed by the monkey's immune system.

Researchers are optimistic and trials in humans will soon begin. The scientists would start by implanting a genetically engineered pig's heart to replace an ailing human heart. It is envisaged that initially the transplant of a pig's heart would only be temporary, keeping a patient alive for weeks or months until a suitable human donor becomes available. This would be followed by a permanent transplant of animal organs once the technique is further refined. It is predicted that the potential market for animal organs used for human transplant would have an annual sales value of more than $1 billion.

Cloning people

Scientists offer cloning as another solution to the problem of supplying suitable organs for transplant. They envisage growing human 'spare parts' from an individual's own cells. To accomplish this, these scientists think they would need just a few human cells; for example, a tiny piece of skin. They would take a human egg cell, remove the nucleus from that cell, and replace it with the nucleus from the individual's skin cell. Having all the new genetic information, the egg cell would then be made to multiply in an artificial womb just as cells do after conception. As a result, the embryo would develop into an individual's identical copy.

The individual's twin would be created early in his or her life, probably around the time of birth. Scientists envisage that the twin would be grown artificially until the beginning of the formation of what would become a brain. This region of latent brain tissue would be removed and destroyed. As a result, the embryo would no longer be human. It would grow in an artificial environment, fed intravenously. At an appropriate stage the twin's growth would be stopped and the twin would be stored. Its organs would become a source for the replacement of any disused, injured or worn out organ for that individual. The twin would be a perfect organ donor since there would be no need for tissue matching and no risk of rejection of the transplanted organ.

Although this seems to be possible only in the distant future, some progress in this direction has already been made. In fact, successful cloning has been shown to be possible in animals. In the early 1960s, John Gurdon, a British scientist, took a frog's egg cell and destroyed its central DNA-bearing structure, that is, its nucleus, so stripping the egg of its own genes. Then the scientist transplanted a nucleus bearing the genes of another frog. The introduced genes masterminded the normal development of the embryo, provided the genes were derived from an embryo.

In 1986, researchers first managed to clone livestock through nuclear transplants derived from an embryo. In 1997, a sheep named "Dolly" was cloned in Scotland.

The major problem is that although our every cell has all the instructions for making a copy of an individual, most of these instructions are 'turned off' and only the ones needed by a particular cell are working. Thus, to accomplish the human cloning envisaged above, scientists would need to find a way to switch on relevant genes.

Nanotechnology

Some scientists believe that significant progress in medicine would be achieved by utilising a technology called nanotechnology. This technology operates on the molecular or nanometre scale. A single nanometre is about the same size as ten atoms together or a thousand times smaller than a micron.

Nanotechnology in medicine aims to create disease-fighting robots (nanorobots) that could work at cellular level. The nanorobots could be responsible for a number of jobs. Some nanorobots are envisaged moving through arteries and removing cholesterol from adjacent walls. Other nanorobots could supplement the immune system by identifying and destroying microscopic invaders. Yet another category of nanorobots could be responsible for cutting away malfunctioning cells such as cancer cells. This would be a truly revolutionary breakthrough in medicine since, except for sudden injuries, most life-threatening emergencies start at microscopic or even submicroscopic level. If doctors, by using nanorobots, could manage to locate and repair minute tissue damage at an early stage, there would be no need for more complicated surgery and the lives of many people could be significantly extended. According to the nanotechnology proponents, this technology could lead to a cure for cancer and could eventually guarantee a biblical life expectancy.

Some scientists argue it will be possible to develop nanotechnology machines in the foreseeable future. K. Eric Drexler, the father of nanotechnology, even predicts that this technology may arrive by 2020. Enthusiasts for nanotechnology point to recent advances in miniaturisation. Toshiba has recently made a transistor which is only 0.04 microns wide—the minimum size of a cell is 1 micron. Finally, researchers have invented the so-called atomic force microscope which can be used to move individual atoms and molecules into new configurations.

Scientists predict that nanomedicine could cost about the same as traditional medicine once research and development costs are paid. Thus, the vision of nanotechnologists may one day become part of everyday life.

Extending lifespan by 200 years

Some scientists believe that in the near future we will be able to extend human lifespan by 200 years or more. This is the case because researchers have recently come to the conclusion that the mechanism responsible for our ageing process is located in each of our body cells. Scientists now understand what keeps a cell's ageing 'clock' running and how to turn it back.

The key to ageing is found in each cell's chromosome which contains tens of thousands of different genes. Each of our chromosomes terminates in regions called telomeres. Each time a cell divides the length of telomeres is reduced. After a number of cell divisions telomeres become too short and the cell dies.

Some types of body cells divide continually and they never age. Examples of such ageless cells are the stem cells in bone marrow which produce blood cells, cancer cells, and the testes that produce sperm. These cells do not age because they have a special enzyme called telomerase that extends the telomere so that the telomeres become long again after cell division, enabling cell replication to continue.

There is a close relationship between the age of the organism and the telomere length of its normal ageing cells. The younger the cells, the longer are the telomeres. Animals which have a short lifespan have short telomeres and those which live longer have long telomeres. When people are getting older their telomeres become shorter and shorter. Children who are born with Hutchinson-Gilford syndrome have a disease which makes them old at birth. We now know that it is caused by very short telomeres. Compared to telomeres in normal children, the telomeres of children with this syndrome are as short as those of a 90-year-old.

The discovery of telomeres has had a profound impact on our ability to extend human life in the near future. Already researchers using a culture of human cells have successfully reset the ageing clock in test tube experiments. The cells, which had a lifespan of 50 divisions, had telomerase added to the cell culture at a time when only five divisions were left before the cells would die. After receiving telomerase, the cells started all over again with another 50 divisions. In this way, these cells lived more than twice as long as normal.

There is great hope that telomerase therapy could also be used to fight cancer. Cancer is a disease in which cells become malignant because they refuse to age and die. This suggests that cancer can be cured by the selective use of telomerase inhibitors. Scientists have already isolated telomerase inhibitors that can prevent the lengthening of telomerases in malignant ovarian cells in vitro. A telomerase inhibitor causes tumour cells to shorten their telomeres and, as a result, these cells age and eventually die. Telomerase inhibitors are currently undergoing trials in animals, but the first human studies are not far off. Some scientists believe that, if research continues at its current rate in the coming years, we will have a cure available to treat most cancers by the year 2005.

Lengthening of telomeres could delay many heart attacks because the cells lining the arteries would be able to divide normally for a longer period of time; this would make them more efficient. However, telomerase therapy would not be able to prevent plaque formation which can close the arteries and cause heart attack. Thus, telomere therapy would make your arteries younger but would not guarantee that they stayed healthy. Hence, we would still have to aim to prevent heart disease by such methods as avoiding cholesterol-containing foods and refraining from smoking. Furthermore, telomerase therapy would do nothing to reverse the damage already done by heart attack or stroke. Moreover, you would still have the same genes that you have now. These set your course for various other diseases so you would still be forced to watch what you eat and take precautions to avoid the many life-shortening factors that have been described in this book.

SELECT BIBLIOGRAPHY

Aldhous P. Rave drug may damage the brain. New Scientist, 1995, Vol. 147, p. 14.

Allard M. Treatment of old age disorders with *Gingko biloba* extract. La Presse Medicale, 1986, Vol. 15, pp. 1540–1545.

Armstrong S.M. and Redman J.R. Melatonin: a chronobiotic with anti-aging properties. Medical Hypotheses, 1991, Vol. 34, pp. 300–309.

Ascherio A. et al. Trans-fatty acids intake and risk of myocardial infarction. Circulation, 1994, Vol. 89, pp. 94–110.

Barry M.D. et al. Possible mechanism of action of (–) deprenyl and other MAO–B inhibitors in some neurologic and psychiatric disorders. Progress in Neurobiology, 1994, Vol. 44, pp. 141–161.

Berkel J. and de Waard, F. Mortality pattern and life expectancy of Seventh-Day Adventists in the Netherlands. International Journal of Epidemiology, 1983, Vol. 12, pp. 455–459.

Bishop J.M. Molecular themes in oncogenesis. Cell, 1991, Vol. 64, pp. 235–248.

Blattner R.J. Comments on current literature: kerosene poisoning. Journal of Pediatrics, 1951, Vol. 39, pp. 391–392.

Bull J.B. et al. The Pyrrolizidine Alkaloids. North-Holland Publishing Co., 1968.

Burr M.L. and Butland, B.K. Heart disease in British vegetarians. American Journal of Clinical Nutrition, 1988, Vol. 48, pp. 830–832.

Candy J.M. et al. Aluminosilicates and senile plaque formation in Alzheimer's Disease. Lancet, 1986, Vol. 1, pp. 354–357.

Caragay A.B. Cancer-preventative foods and ingredients. Food Technology, 1992, Vol. 46, pp. 65–68.

Carrol K.K. Review of clinical studies on cholesterol lowering response to soy protein. Journal of the American Dietetics Association, 1991, Vol. 91, pp. 820–827.

Celermayer D.S. et al. Passive smoking and impaired endothelium dependant arterial dilatation in healthy young adults. New England Journal of Medicine, 1996, Vol. 334, pp. 150–154.

Cerda J.J. et al. The effects of grapefruit pectin in patients at risk for coronory heart disease without altering diet or lifestyle. Clinical Cardiology, 1988, Vol. 11, pp. 588–594.

Cheng H.H. et al. The antitumour effect of cultivated *Ganoderma lucidum* extract. Journal of Chinese Oncology Society, 1982, Vol. 1, pp. 12–16.

Chihara G. et al. Fractionation and purification of the polysaccharides with marked anti-tumour activity especially lentinan, from *Lentinus edodes* (an edible mushroom). Cancer Research, 1980, Vol. 30, pp. 2776–2781.

Cristol R. Rester jeune à tout age: myth au réalité. Hachette, Paris, 1993.

Culver K.W. Gene Therapy. A Handbook for Physicians. Liebert Mary Ann Inc., 1994.

Cutler R.G. Antioxidants and aging. American Journal of Clinical Nutrition, 1991, Vol. 53, pp. 373–379.

Durham W.F and Williams C.H. Mutagenic, teratogenic, and carcinogenic properties of pesticides. Annual Review of Entomology, 1972, Vol. 17, pp. 123–148.

Evans I.A. et al. Carcinogenic activity of bracken. Nature, 1965, Vol. 208, pp. 913–914.

Flood J.F., Smith G.E. and Roberts E. Dehydroepiandrosterone and its sulphate enchance memory retention in mice. Brain Research, 1988, Vol. 447, pp. 267–268.

Friedman T.A. A brief history of gene therapy. National Genetics, 1992, Vol. 2, pp. 93–98.

Ganrot P.O. Metabolism and possible health effects of aluminium. Environmental Health Perspectives, 1986, Vol. 65, pp. 363–418.

Gessner B. et al. Study of the longterm action of *Ginko biloba* extract on vigillance and mental performance as determined by means of quantitative pharmaco-EEG and psychometric measurements. Arzneimittelforschung, 1985, Vol. 35, pp. 1459–1465.

Gibbs J.B. and Oliff A. A pharmaceutic research in molecular oncology. Cell, 1994, Vol. 79, pp. 193–198.

Gillman M.W. et al. Protective effect of fruits and vegetables on development of stroke in men. Journal of the American Medical Association, 1995, Vol. 273, pp. 1113–1117.

Goldberg A. et al. Soybean protein independently lowers plasma cholesterol levels in primary hypercholesterolemia. Atherosclerosis, 1982, Vol. 43, pp. 355–368.

Haber D.A. Telomeres, cancer and immortality. New England Journal of Medicine, 1995, Vol. 332, pp. 955–956.

Hartwell L.H . and Kasten M.B. Cell cycle control and cancer. Science, 1994, Vol. 266, pp. 1821–1828.

Hinds P.W. and Weinberg R.A. Tumor suppressor genes. Current Opinion in Genetics and Development, 1994, Vol. 4, pp. 135–141.

Hirono I. Carcinogenic principles isolated from bracken fern. CRC Critical Review in Toxicology, 1986, Vol. 17, pp. 1–11.

Hirono I. et al. Carcinogenic activity of coltsfoot *Tussilago farfara L.* Gann, 1976, Vol. 67, pp. 125–129.

Hocman G. Prevention of cancer: vegetables and plants. Comparative Biochemistry and Physiology, 1989, Vol. 93B, pp. 201–212.

Hopgood F. The really little engines that might. Technology Review, 1993, Vol. 96, pp. 30–37.

Houghton P. Herbal products. Gingko. The Pharmaceutical Journal, 1994, Vol. 253, pp. 122–123.

Ishiuama T., Morita Y. and Toyama S.A. A clinical study of the effect of coenzyme Q on congestive heart failure. Japanese Heart Journal, 1976, Vol. 17, pp. 32–36.

Jain A.K. et al. Can garlic reduce levels of serum lipids? A controlled study. American Journal of Medicine, 1993, Vol. 94, pp. 632–635.

Joosten E. et al. Metabolic evidence that deficiencies of vitamin B_{12} (cobalamin), folate and vitamin B_6 occur commonly in elderly people. American Journal of Clinical Nutrition, 1993, Vol. 58, pp. 468–476.

Kelly S.P. Aconite poisoning. Medical Journal of Australia, 1990, Vol. 153, p. 449.

Kleijnen J. and Knipschild P. *Gingko biloba*. Lancet, 1992, Vol. 340, pp. 1136–1139.

Komori A. et al. Anticarcinogenic activity of green tea polyphenols. Japanese Journal of Clinical Oncology, 1993, Jun. 23, pp. 186–190.

Larrick J.W. and Burck K.L. Gene Therapy: Application of Molecular Biology. Elsevier, 1991.

Langer R. and Vacanti J.P. Tissue engineering. Science, 1993, Vol. 260, pp. 920–926.

Lewis H.D. Jr. et al. Protective effects of aspirin against acute myocardial infarction and death in men with unstable angina: results of a veterans administration cooperative study. New England Journal of Medicine, 1983, Vol. 309, pp. 396–403.

Loria R.M. et al. Protection against acute lethal virus infection with the native steroid dehydroepiandrosterone (DHEA). Journal of Medical Virology, 1988, Vol. 26, pp. 301–314.

Luthy J. et al. Pyrrolizidine alkaloid in arzneipflanzen der Boraginaceen: *Borago officinalis L.* and *Pulmonaria officinalis L.* Pharmaceutica Acta Helvetiae, 1984, Vol. 59, pp. 242–246.

Macek K. East meets West to balance immunologic yin and yan. Journal of the American Medical Association, 1984, Vol. 251, pp. 433–441.

Masoro E.J. Dietary restriction and aging. Journal of the American Geriatrics Society, 1993, Vo. 41, pp. 993–999.

Melville A. and Johnson C. Cured to Death, The Effects of Prescription Drugs. Angus and Robertson, 1982.

Messina M. and Messina V. Increasing use of soyfoods and their potential role in cancer prevention. Journal of the American Dietetics Association, 1991, Vol. 91, pp. 836–840.

Moller J.O. Cancer risk among Danish male Seventh-Day Adventists and other temperance society members. Journal of the National Cancer Institute, 1983, Vol. 70, pp. 1011–1014.

Mooney D.J., Organ G., Valanti J. and Langer R. Design and fabrication of biodegradable polymer devices to engineer tubular tissues. Cell Transplantation, 1994, Vol. 3, pp. 203–210.

Morgan K. et al. Customary physical activity, psychological wellbeing and successful aging. Aging and Society, 1991, Vol. 11, pp. 399–415.

Mulligan R.C. The basic science of gene therapy. Science, 1993, Vol. 260, pp. 926–932.

Nakamura Y. et al. Protection of ischemic myocardium with coenzyme Q_{10}. Cardiovascular Research, 1982, Vol. 16, pp. 132–137.

Negri E. et al. Vegetable and fruit consumption and cancer risk. International Journal of Cancer, 1994, Vol. 48, pp. 350–354.

Nuovo J. Use of dietary fibre to lower cholesterol, American Family Physician, 1989, Vol. 39, pp. 137–140.

Oden M. Prolongation of the life span in rats. Journal of the American Geriatrics Society, 1973, Vol. 21, pp. 450–451.

Olsen E.J. et al. Gerovital–H3: a clinical trial as an antidepressant. Journal of Gerontology, 1978, Vol. 33, pp. 514–520.

Ornish D. et al. Can lifestyle changes reverse coronary heart disease? The lifestyle heart trial. Lancet, 1990, Vol. 336, pp. 624–626.

Osfeld A., Smith C.M. and Stotsky B.A. The systemic use of procaine in the treatment of the elderly: a review. Journal of the American Geriatrics Society, 1977, Vol. 25, pp. 1–19.

Packer L. Protective role of viamin E in biological systems. American Journal of Clinical Nutrition, 1991, Vol. 53, pp 1050S–1055S.

Paffenbarger R.S. et al. Physical activity, all-cause mortality and longevity of College alumni. New England Journal of Medicine, 1986, Vol. 314, pp. 605–613.

Penn N.D. et al. The effects of dietary supplementation with vitamins A, C and E on cell-mediated immune function in elderly long-stay patients: a randomised controlled trial. Age and Ageing, 1991, Vol. 20, pp. 169–174.

Perchellet J.P. et al. Antitumour-promoting activities of tannic acid, ellagic acid and several gallic acid derivatives in mouse skin. Basic Life Science, 1992, Vol. 59, pp. 783–801.

Perl D.P. and Brody A.R. Alzheimer's disease: x-ray spectronometric evidence of aluminium accumulation in neurofibrillary tangle-bearing neurons. Science, 1980, Vol. 208, pp. 297–299.

Peto R. et al. Can dietary beta-carotene materially reduce human cancer rates? Nature, 1981, Vol. 290, pp. 201–207.

Ridker M.P. et al. Comfrey tea and hepatic veno-occlusive disease. Lancet, 1989, Vol. 1, pp. 657–658.

Saito H., Yoshida Y. and Takagi K. Effects of *Panax ginseng* root on exhaustive exercise in mice. Japanese Journal of Pharmacology, 1974, Vol. 24, pp. 119–127.

Salonen J.T. Association between serum selenium and the risk of cancer. American Journal of Epidemiology, 1984, Vol. 120, pp. 342–349.

SALT Collaborative Group Swedish Aspirin Low-Dose Trial of 75 mg aspirin as secondary prophylaxis after cerebrovascular ischaemic events. Lancet, 1991, Vol. 338, pp. 1345–1349.

Schmidt, K. Antioxidant vitamins and B-carotene: effects on immunocompetence. American Journal of Clinical Nutrition, 1991, Vol. 53, pp. 383S–385S.

Segelman A.B. et al. Sassafras and herb tea: potential health hazards. Journal of the American Medical Association, 1976, Vol. 236, p. 477.

Sharma O.P. et al. Soy of dietary source plays a preventive role against the pathogenesis of prostatitis. Journal of Steroid Biochemical Molecular Biology, 1992, Vol. 43, pp. 557–564.

Skolnick A.A. Cancer cells' immortality may prove their undoing. Journal of the American Medical Association, 1995, Vol. 273, pp. 1247–1248.

Tagaki K., Saito H. and Nababa H. Pharmaceutical studies of *Panax ginseng* root. Japanese Journal of Pharmacology, 1972, Vol. 22, pp. 245–259.

Talalaj S. and Czechowicz A.S. Herbal Remedies: Harmful and Beneficial Effects. Hill of Content, 1989.

Truswell A.S. ABC of nutrition. Adults young and old. British Medical Journal, 1985, Vol. 29, pp. 466–469.

United States Preventive Services Task Force. Aspirin prophylaxis for cardiovascular disease. American Family Physician, 1989, Vol. 40, pp. 117–120.

Vanherweghem J.L. et al. Rapidly progressive interstitial renal fibrosis in young women: association with slimming regimen including Chinese herbs. Lancet, 1993, Vol. 341, pp. 387–391.

Vitamin E supplementation enhances immune response in the elderly. Nutrition Review, 1992, Vol. 50, pp. 85–87.

Wahlquist M.L. et al. Food and Health. Issues and Directions. John Libbey, 1987.

Walter S. et al. The association of cutaneous malignant melanoma and fluorescent light exposure. American Journal of Epidemiology, 1992, Vol. 135, pp. 749–762.

Weidruch R. and Walford R.L. Life span and spontaneous cancer incidence in mice dietary restricted beginning one year of age. Science, 1982, Vol. 215, pp. 1415–1418.

Yang P. and Banwell J.G. Dietary fibre: its role in the pathogenesis and treatment of constipation. Practical Gastroenterology, 1986, Vol. 6, pp. 28–32.

Yu B.P. (ed.) Modulation of Aging Processes by Dietary Restriction. CRS Press, 1994.

Yu S.Y. et al. Regional variation of cancer mortality incidence and its relation to selenium levels in China. Biological Trace Elements Research, 1985, Vol. 7, pp. 21–29.

Ziegler R. G. Vegetables, fruits and carotenoids and the risk of cancer. American Journal of Clinical Nutrition, 1991, Vol. 53, pp. 251S–259S.

INDEX